dedication

My Parents
You rock. I am forever grateful
for your love, guidance and support.

My Son
I am so proud of the man you
have become. Keep pushing Tiny.

All of the Home Cooks
Get ready to learn just how good
healthy living can be.

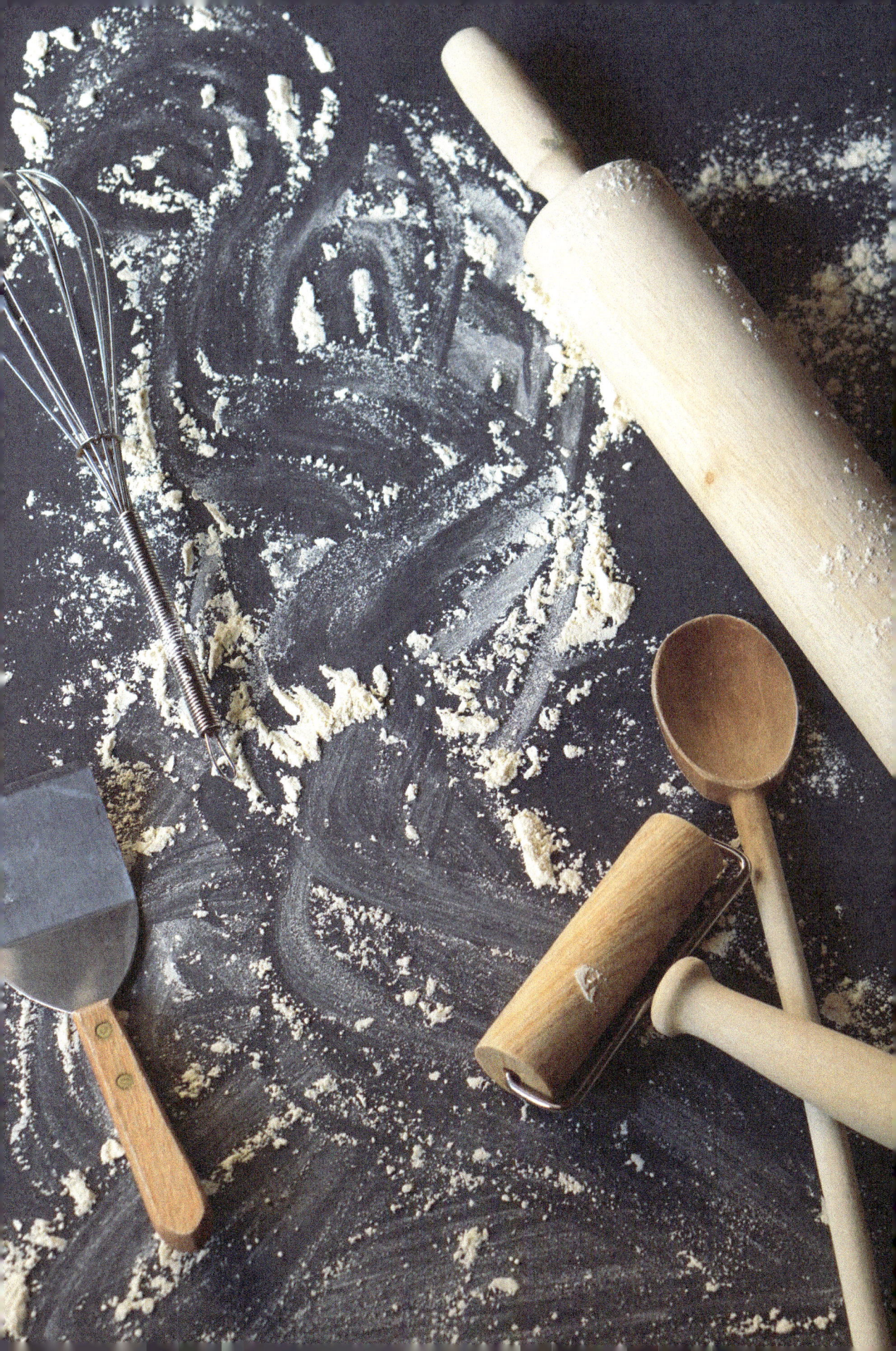

Healthy Bites
for the
Mind, Body & Soul

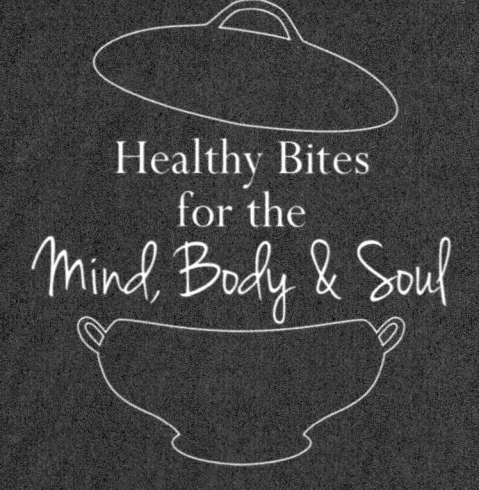

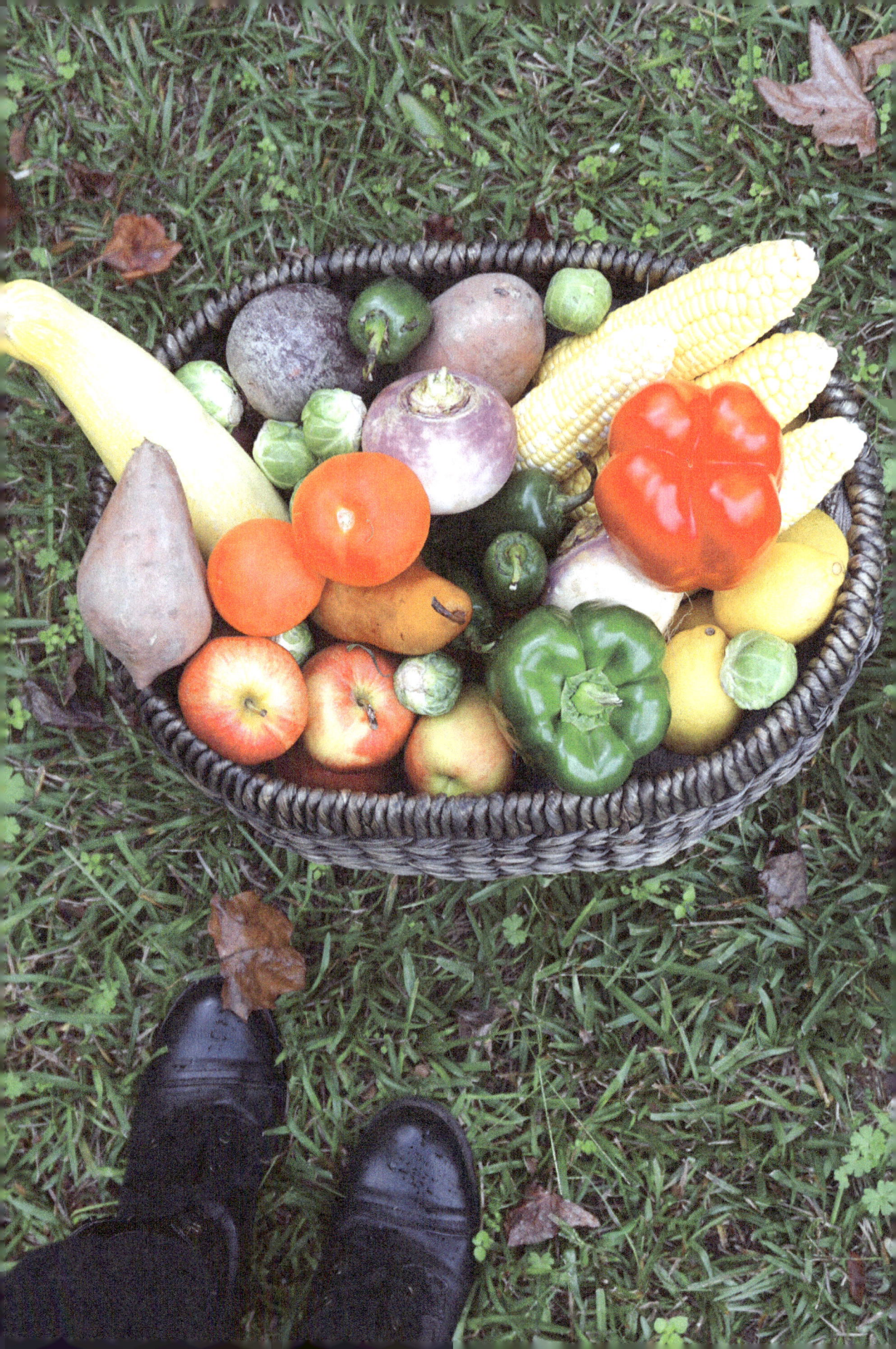

Healthy Bites for the Mind, Body & Soul

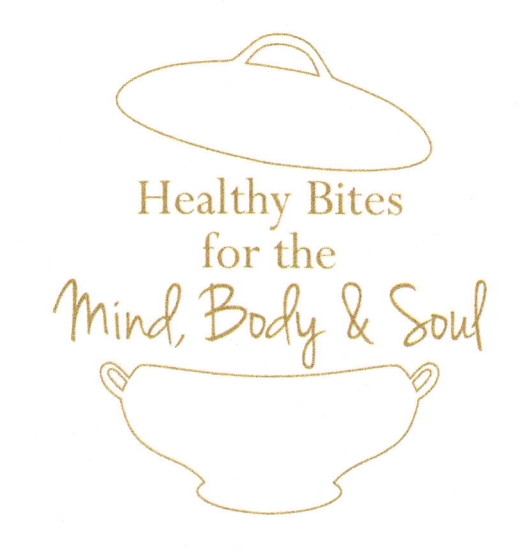

Over 50 recipes that are inspired for healthier living

Sugar free.
Gluten free.
(Mostly) Dairy free.

RECIPES + FOOD PHOTOGRAPHY BY
PATRICE L. JOHNSON

All rights reserved. No part of this publication may be reproduced in any form or by any means, including scanning, photocopying or otherwise, without the prior written consent of the publisher.

© 2017 Patrice L. Johnson.

Printed and bound in the
United States of America.

Printed by IngramSpark

Book Design by Patrice L. Johnson, Virtual Illustrations.
Food photography by Patrice L. Johnson.
Food styling by Patrice L. Johnson.

Edited by Annetta Watkins-Foard.

Photo credits: Contents (Maksim Shebeko/Fotolia), p.45 (bhofack2/123RF), p. 141 (Daffodilred/fotolia), p. 145 (studiograndouest/123RF)

This book is not intended to be a substitute for professional medical advice. The author and publisher disclaim any and all liability arising directly or indirectly from the use of any information contained in this book. Please consult a health professional about specifics regarding your health concerns. In the instance that a particular brand is mentioned in this publication, it does not imply endorsement by the company.

ISBN -13: 978-0-692-86964-2 hardcover

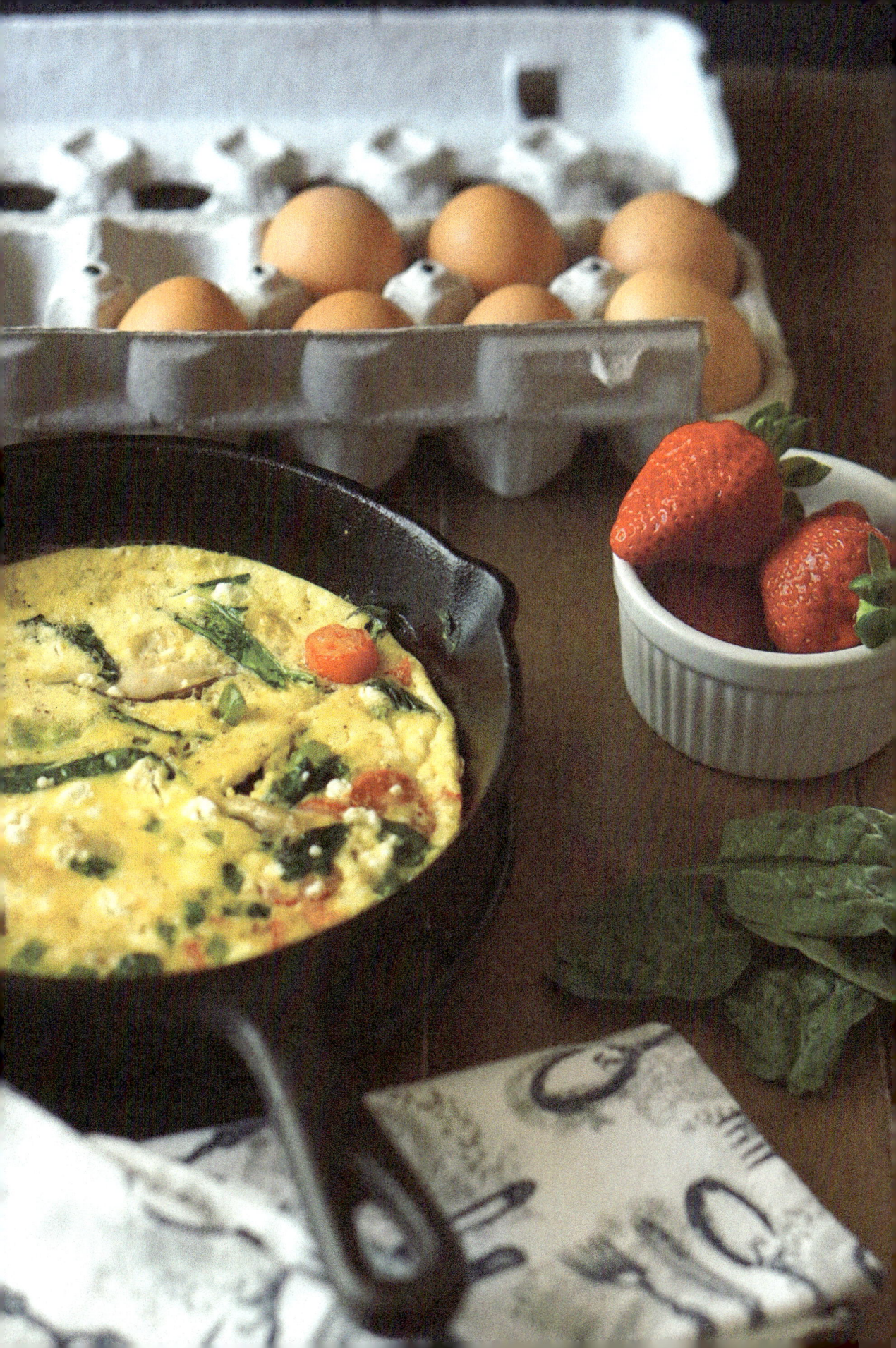

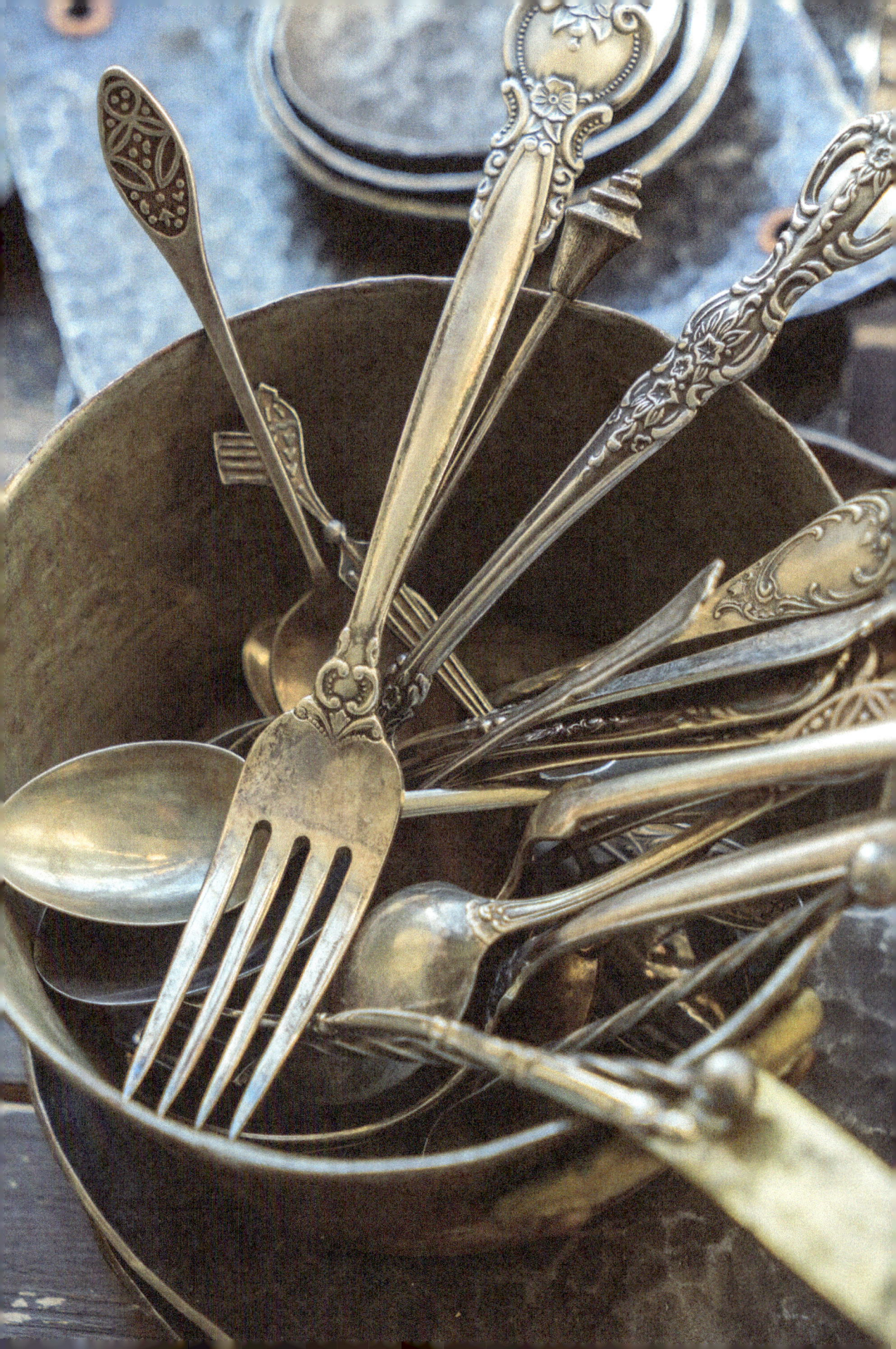

- contents -

p. 1
Introduction
Why I started eating healthier and why you should too!

p. 21
Breakfast
Start the most important meal of the day with one of these healthy, hearty dishes.

p. 47
Lunch and Mains
Quick and easy meals for a dinner that will wow your guests, even those who are not eating healthy.

p. 87
Sides 'n Such
Vegetables, side dishes and easy snack ideas.

p. 105
Desserts
Dessert does not have to be a thing of the past once you commit to eating healthy.

p. 117
Beverages
Detox, cool off on a summer day, or simply nourish your body with these healthy, nutrient-packed juices and teas.

p. 133
Condiments
Say no to store-bought! Make your own condiments at home.

p. 141
A Couple o' Extras

> no one is *born*
> a great cook, one learns
> by *doing*
> — Julia Child

introduction

    I am not sure where my love of cooking began but I remember fondly sitting at the kitchen table, as a child, with my grandmother while she baked homemade cinnamon rolls or dipped her homemade cornbread in buttermilk and savored every bite. She was a great cook and an excellent baker. Nana always had a pound cake or coconut cake in the fridge and there was never a shortage of leftovers at her house. Perhaps that is where I developed a passion for food. But eventually I, too, was known for having a good Southern cooked meal and a few desserts or frozen treats in the house.

    My desserts were so popular amongst my friends and family that they convinced me to start blogging. I enjoyed doing blogging immensely; but it was time consuming and I would later change my diet. So I could no longer promote those unhealthy, albeit delicious, desserts, baked goods and pasta dishes as I had before.

    I initially ended up changing my diet to avoid ever having to take conventional medicine again and have learned how healing foods can boost the immune system, cure many ailments and prevent disease and poor health. I later learned that I had a chronic illness so I have become even more strict about what I eat and there is no such thing as a cheat day. I know. Sad, right? However, my meals are nutritious, delicious and packed with flavor! My decision to write this book came from a desire to help others treat their bodies naturally and be more conscious about the foods we consume. I also want others to see how easy it is to cook from scratch so you know what is in the food you eat and can discontinue eating these sugary, fatty, unhealthy foods.

    Don't let the plating discourage you. Most of these dishes are easy to make and the ingredients can be found at your local farmer's market or just about any grocery store, not just the high-end stores.

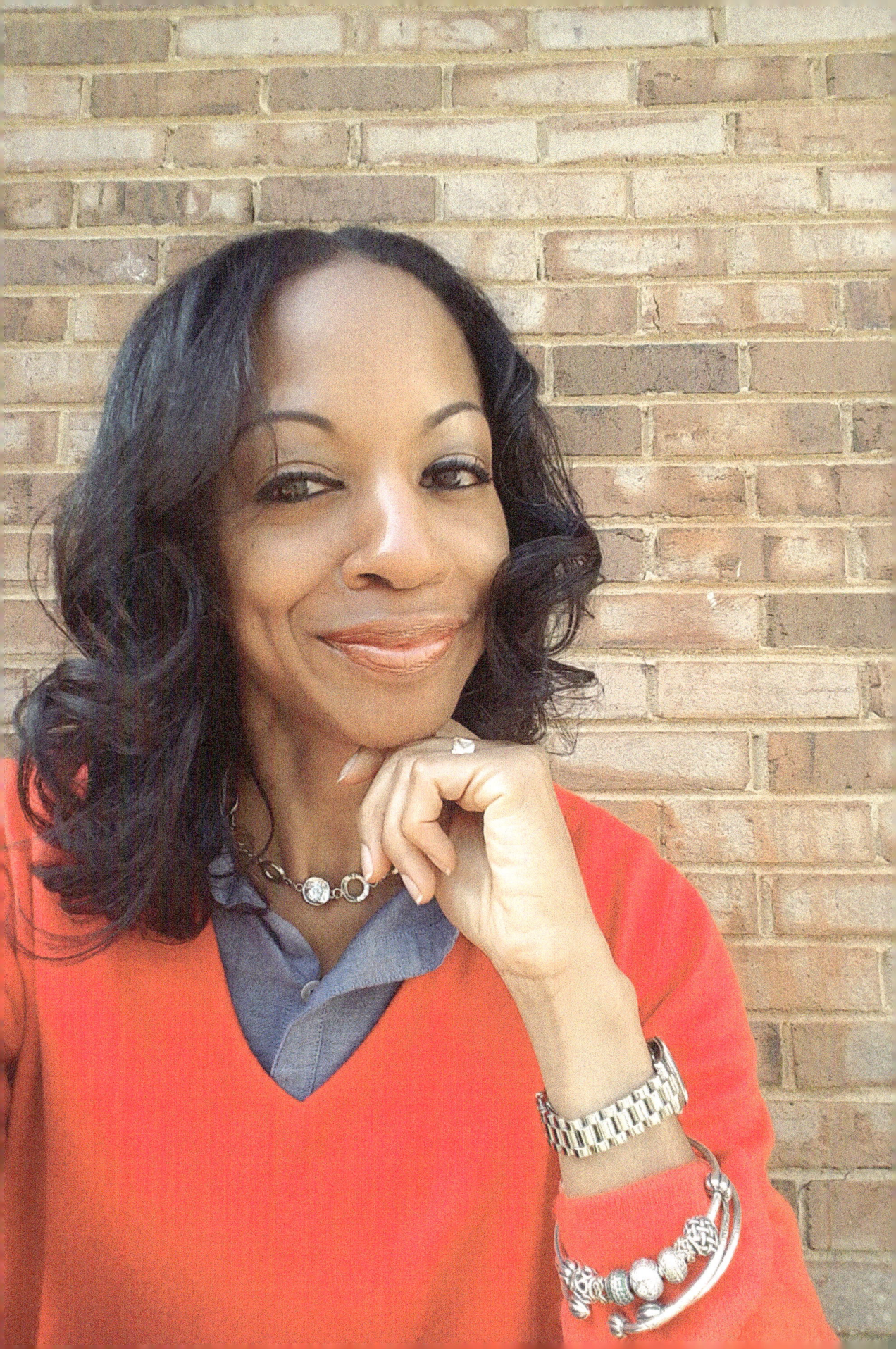

skinny gal

I was always the skinny girl. So I never got bogged down with calorie consumption, dieting or eating healthy. But, once I got in my late 20's, I began these frequent trips to the doctor's office with a host of unexplained illnesses that I later learned were likely signs of me having Lyme Disease, which I contracted sometime around 1993. While I had been sick over the years, it was not until 2013 that I became extremely ill. I would later learn that my weakened immune system (due to diet, toxins and heavy antibiotic use) may have triggered the disease to rear its ugly head and begin to flourish.

Some of the issues I consistently had were sinus, kidney, bladder and respiratory infections. I was typically prescribed an antibiotic for a two-week span, which began a vicious cycle. Due to my heavy consumption of dairy products and sugar, that continually led to a lot of mucus production, congestion, and yeast overgrowth. I would take the prescribed antibiotic. It would further suppress my immune system. I would continue eating sweets and dairy, which were feeding the yeast and causing mucus; so as soon as I would finish the course of antibiotics, I would need another one or need to be switched to a stronger prescription - because I was developing an immunity to certain antibiotics.

In October of 2010, I became ill and ended up in the hospital and was diagnosed with clostridium difficile (c.diff), the most serious cause of antibiotic-associated diarrhea that can lead to a severe inflammation of the colon, often resulting from an imbalance of the normal gut flora by antibiotics. Over time, my poor diet and antibiotic overuse began to weaken my immune system and I had a serious overgrowth of negative flora or bad bacteria. I was told that c. diff was contagious and that there was a possibility that I would be quarantined. And the one thing that the attendant made sure to emphasize was that I should be cautious about taking another antibiotic again.

Antibiotics definitely kill the bad bacteria in your system, which is a benefit. But the harm is that they also kill all of the good bacteria. If you do not take a probiotic, along with the antibiotic, to replenish the good bacteria, it can deplete your immune system, taking years for your body to be restored to normalcy. Since I was taking at least two antibiotics a month to treat my sinus and respiratory issues, my system never had a chance to recover.

So I left the hospital, determined to be prepared for what would happen the next time I got sick and could no longer rely on an antibiotic for treatment. As I began to read about c. diff and what caused it, I also began to see that several other ailments I had might have been tied into the disease. One of those would be Candida. Most people relate Candida to the bacteria that causes yeast infections. What they do not know is that it can also be systemic and cause a host of problems in both males and females. Almost everyone has Candida Albicans in their gut, but some may also have Candidiasis, an overgrowth of Candida, which can be caused by taking too many antibiotics, having a diet rich in sugar and carbs and stress. I had all of the above. I started to see a pattern here. Antibiotics. Poor diet. Bacteria. Toxins. Intestinal Health. These words were in almost every article I read on my fact-finding journey.

From that point on, I became obsessed with gaining knowledge about how to change my lifestyle - my diet, my exercise regimen and...my number of trips to the doctor and hospital.

I eventually came to terms with the fact that I was going to have to drastically change my diet. In 2010, during the holiday season, I had a Girl's Night In at my place. I had every dessert you could imagine, but as I prepared those desserts I knew that I could not enjoy them with the knowledge I now had about the correlation with diet and my poor health. That night was a turning point for me as I decided then to never consume sugar again. That was the first step in my journey towards healthier eating. I have a close girlfriend whose small children were eating hummus and foods I had never heard of at that time, using baking soda for deodorant, making their own skin products...and she told me that I should consider doing a detox to cleanse my body, before starting on this sugar-free journey. Of course I read up on that too and decided to give it a whirl. I started off doing a cleanse at the first of the year and, at the instruction of the health food store personnel, did a Candida cleanse first and then a total body detox. That was a doozy! Since I had never done a cleanse before and had been eating any and every thing I ever wanted, I had no idea that my body was so toxic. For those who have never cleansed before, the more toxic your body is, the more intense going through a detox will be.

Toxins are everywhere - in the water we drink, in the air we breathe, the chemicals and products we use, the foods we consume...our bodies are constantly using energy to fight those toxins and rebuild body tissue and they can affect our overall health and wellness.

A lot of people argue that a cleanse is not needed and that your body can do all of the necessary things to detox, without the help of natural herbs and medicines. However, in my experience, a cleanse has helped me with better digestion, improved my sleeping patterns, cleared my skin, regulated my bowels, rejuvenated and gave me more energy, reduced bloating around my midsection, cleared my sinuses, and much more.

Some of the signs that you may need to cleanse are constant fatigue, frequent headaches, frequent constipation, body aches, foul smelling bowels, acne, dark circles under your eyes, bad breath, frequent heartburn, constant bloating, postnasal drip, excessive sinus issues, itchy skin, rashes...the list goes on.

The first few days of any cleanse can be rough as you are going through what is called the Herxheimer Reaction. This period is where you feel worse before you get better, but it is a signal that the detox is working as it should be. Once the toxins begin to flood your bloodstream, you get the initial period of feeling sick. During the Herxheimer Reaction, one may experience chills, get symptoms that resemble the flu, get rashes, have worsened headaches, etc. but there are many things that you can do to alleviate those issues or speed them along. You can choose to detox with supplements. Or you can try milder versions of detoxing like sweating toxins out at a sauna or with a detox bath, or by juicing. I will share some of my favorite detox remedies and juices that are a gentler method of cleansing the liver and the kidneys.

Once my detoxing was completed, I was ready to start with a clean eating regimen. This part was not too hard for me since I cooked every day and made most of what I ate from scratch. My new diet mainly consisted of chicken, fish, turkey, fresh vegetables, fruits, and honey and stevia for sweeteners. Nothing was going to keep me from eating well if that meant I could eliminate going to the doctor and taking antibiotics.

Substitutions for some of the foods you should eliminate with a clean(er) diet

AVOID	SUBSTITUTE
Processed Sugar	Stevia or Wild/Raw Honey
Cheese	Goat Cheese, Vegan Cheese Alternatives (Soy-free)
Margarine	Butter, Ghee, Coconut oil
Cow's Milk	Coconut milk, Almond milk, Quinoa milk, Cashew milk, Rice milk
Cooking Oil	Coconut oil (high heat), olive oil
Soy Sauce	Coconut Aminos
White rice	Brown rice, Cauliflower "rice", Quinoa
Grits	Polenta (if corn products are allowed)
Whipped cream	Whipped coconut cream
Peanut butter	Almond butter, Cashew butter
Extracts/flavoring	Alcohol-free extracts, Flavored Stevia
Cornstarch	Arrowroot starch
Whey protein	Pea protein, plant-based protein powder
Buttermilk	Alternative milk (almond, rice, quinoa or coconut) + 1 tablespoon of organic apple cider vinegar to sour milk or lemon juice
White Flour	Gluten free flour blend, Brown rice flour, Almond flour, Sorghum flour, Buckwheat flour, Quinoa flour, Garbanzo bean flour

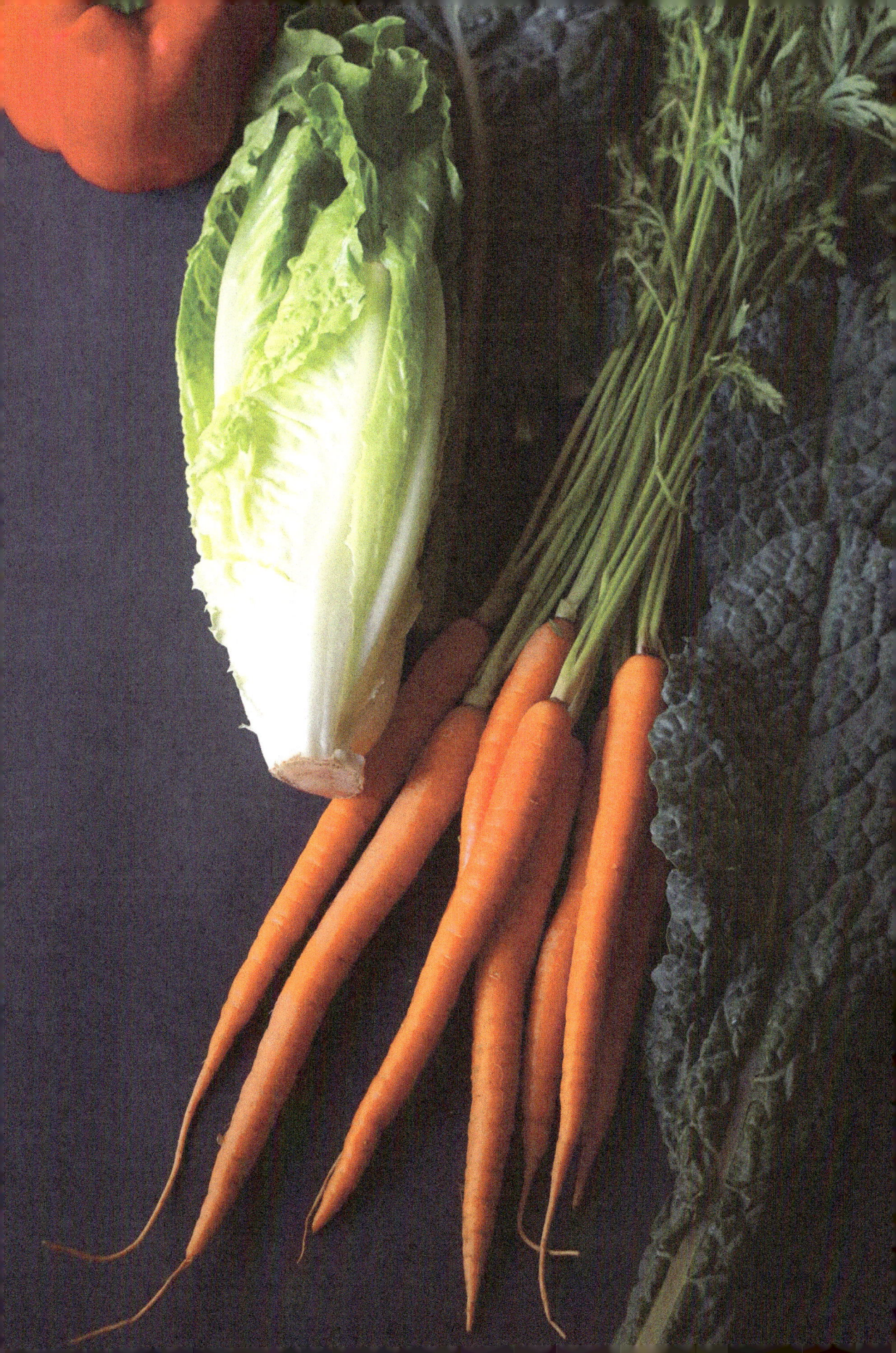

let's get clean

So what do you eat when you make the decision to eat healthier? And what does eating clean really mean? Eating clean is basically eating more raw, whole and unprocessed foods. Eating foods in its most natural state. I ate fruits and vegetables all the time but I was eating a lot of dried fruits, which were loaded with sugar, and a lot of vegetables that were in the can, which were loaded with sodium. I realized that I needed to be eating raw, organic and lightly steamed vegetables to truly get the nutritional benefits from them. And for me, since sugar was also feeding the Candida, I needed to cut out all forms of sugar, not just dessert.

Sugar is in almost everything on the shelves. So it became very important to learn how to read labels. When you are checking labels for sugar content, look for things like:

- White sugar
- Corn syrup
- Molasses
- Dextrose
- Turbinado
- High Fructose Corn Syrup
- Processed Fructose
- Sucrose

With that said, if sugar is in almost everything you can buy, that means that I had to begin to truly make everything I consumed from scratch, down to the condiments. That also makes it extremely hard to enjoy a nice dinner out with friends, because you really have no idea how foods are being prepared.

In addition, I eliminated dairy from my diet and began to use hemp, rice, almond and coconut milk. I eliminated cheese altogether but have since added goat cheese into my diet. If you crave mozzarella, pepper jack or cheddar cheese, there are some fairly decent cheese alternatives on the market, such as Daiya and Vegan Gourmet, that are a pretty good substitute for cheese lovers.

I did this for a few months and quickly got bored with this clean eating stuff. In 2010, there was just not as much variety as there is now for folks who are trying to eat healthier. So I soon became determined to learn a way to enjoy all of the foods I ate before, but with healthier ingredients. Otherwise, I could not imagine continuing this journey for a significant amount of time.

I started to read about organic foods, gluten vs. cooking with alternative flours; cage free vs. battery cage, wild vs. farm raised, whole wheat vs. whole grain; soy vs. almond, hemp and coconut milk.

And then I began to learn why they cook differently and started to experiment with my favorite dishes.

I continued down this path for almost two years without even a trip to the doctor's office. I was so excited that this clean eating regimen was really working.

I came across a lot of skeptics along the way but no matter what people said, I knew I was feeling better and was looking fit. I started working out in the gym five days a week and was putting on weight.

Life was good.

...until the day I decided to start on a multi-vitamin that was really large in size. I have trouble swallowing large pills, but had been doing pretty well with my supplements so I figured this one would not be too bad either. However, the day after starting the multi-vitamin, I started having trouble breathing and swallowing. The food that I was chewing was coming back up through my esophagus and causing me to choke. After not being able to get anyone on the telephone, I called 911. But by that time, I was lying in my bathroom floor, unable to breathe and having spasms.

I was able to get to my front door to allow the EMTs to enter. They put me on oxygen and began to ask several questions about what was going on. They were under the impression that I was having a heart attack.

Although I am no doctor, I felt very strongly that what I was experiencing was not a heart attack. And because I had dealt with so much chest pain in the past, I felt like I knew what symptoms to be on the lookout for with a heart attack. I continued to explain to them that I had taken a pill the night before and that it felt, to me, that the pill was lodged in my throat. Considering the fact that I drink 10-12 cups of water daily, they did not feel that this was possible.

Upon rushing me to the hospital I was treated for a heart attack in spite of my protests. I was given nitroglycerine, morphine and some other potent drugs after being admitted to the hospital. After having no relief from the chest pain upon taking the nitroglycerine, they deduced that my pains were not from a heart attack. I still insisted that the pill was somehow the culprit. But as usual, no one was listening.

Eventually, the doctor said she was out of options and would allow me to stay overnight to see a Gastroenterologist the next day. When the doctor came in and performed the endoscopy, it was determined that the pill had not actually remained in my esophagus but remnants of the pill burned a hole in my esophagus and now I had an ulcer.

After being given several medications during my stay, I was also put on a high dosage of proton pump inhibitors (PPIs) to heal the ulcer for an 8-week duration. After two years of not even having a sinus infection that I could not cure naturally, I was now back to square one. In that short period of time, the drugs suppressed my immune system and rendered my body toxic again.

It became very discouraging that one visit could cause a setback; but my immune system was so weak that after being "clean" for almost two years, this onslaught of medicine was more than my body could handle.

I now knew enough about toxins, after studying over the last few years, to know that I may need to detox my body again. But during the 8 weeks of taking the drugs to heal the ulcer, I began to go through a myriad of aches and pains - leg pains, body aches, fatigue, chest pains. The doctor dismissed all of these things and said they had nothing to do with the medication.

So back to the computer I went. I was learning that I really had to be my own advocate and my own medical detective.

I tried various things to restore myself to good health but I still never got back to feeling as good as I had prior to the multi-vitamin incident.

2 steps forward...10 steps back

I continued to work towards getting back to the old me. I started back on my workout regimen and things were turning around. And then in January of 2013 my girlfriend and I headed to the gym for our early evening workout and I started feeling sick. It was the kind of sick where you feel like you are just lifting too much without enough protein. So I told her I was going to head home and would see her the next day. But I have not stepped back in the gym since that evening.

When I got home, I showered and ate, and I felt like things were a little off but nothing I could put my finger on. The next day I could barely walk or get out of bed, which was odd because we had not worked out our legs the day prior. I went about my normal day and drove to a few meetings but started having a feeling of weakness on the entire right side of my body. It was a little more severe than any of the usual weakness I had experienced in years prior.

I attempted to ignore it but was having trouble keeping my balance and was having blurred vision. I stopped by the hospital on the way home from a meeting and explained my symptoms to them. The doctor on duty told me that it was unusual to have pain that was on one side only, unless you were having a stroke. They ruled out a stroke or a heart attack and sent me home to rest. The next day, I still could not get it together and ended up back at the hospital. They did some additional testing and the doctor suggested that perhaps

I had the early stages of an autoimmune disease. We have a history of Multiple Sclerosis (MS) in our family. So I went home and started looking up autoimmune diseases and found that almost every symptom they had in the articles I read, was a symptom I had been experiencing.

In the coming weeks, the weakness in my right side got much worse, I still had trouble with my eyesight, I became sensitive to light, could not keep my balance, had swollen lymph nodes, neck pains, jaw pains, TMJ, headache, blurry vision, tingling, insomnia, fatigue, shortness of breath, itchy eyes, rashes, chills, fullness in neck, nausea, constipation, numbness, uncontrollable tremors, itching all over my body with no rash present, and considerable weight loss. I was only around 124 lbs to start with, most of which was muscle weight I'd gained through strength training at the gym.

I started obsessing about the weight after looking at a photo posted on social media and seeing how thin I looked. So I then began to weigh myself every day and the weight just kept coming off. In three months, I went from 124 to 109.2. I still could not fathom that I might have some sort of chronic disease. But it was becoming apparent that my life, as I had previously known it, was changing. My pains were so bad that I was unable to drive and even make it from the bed on some days. How could I have gone from lifting weights and being healthy to being bedridden almost overnight?

In the weeks to come, I saw several doctors, made numerous hospital trips and was told that it did seem as though I had an autoimmune disease but that they are hard to detect until they are upon you. I might be getting signals that something was going wrong but it may be in the early stages. If this was the early stages, I certainly did not want to see what this disease might look like full out. Some of the diseases mentioned were fibromyalgia, MS, Lupus, Crohn's and ALS. I was referred to a neurologist but it would be months before I was able to get in to see the doctor. So I sat in pain and waited to get in to the specialist.

So many things were running through my mind. Being confined to one room gives you a lot of time to think. How could I convince others to eat healthy and change their lifestyle if I am eating clean and working out and suddenly sick and bedridden? Will I ever be able to drive again? I use my hands for work, how will I work if I can't even lift my arms? Will I have to give up living alone and move in with someone so that I have a caregiver around the clock? Will I ever work out again? Cook a meal?

I knew that many diseases can be seen through the eyes so I made an appointment to see my eye doctor, since I was in limbo until my appointment with the neurologist. In addition to the concern I had about MS or some autoimmune disease, I was beginning to have a lot of trouble with blurred vision and photophobia (sensitivity to light).

When I visited my eye doctor he asked about my symptoms and he, too, said that most of those pointed to an autoimmune disorder. But he did not find anything that pointed to that in my eye exams. He repeated, as the hospital doctor had, that autoimmune diseases sometimes take a while to show up, so I may have to be my own best advocate. If I did not get the answers from one doctor, I would need to try again.

So the day finally came where I was able to visit the neurologist. Now I must admit, because of my previous experiences with doctors being dismissive, I had a lot of negative feelings about seeing this neurologist. And this visit was no exception. During the visits to the hospital, because of my symptoms, the doctors did a basic cognitive test. You know the one where they take the hammer and hit your knee...have you follow their finger to see if you respond accordingly? I had done that several times during the weeks leading up to my appointment with the specialist. So my expectations of this visit were to be scheduled for an MRI and see what was causing these issues. She performed the same basic cognitive test and then told me I did not have MS and she did not feel as though an MRI would be necessary. She basically sent me home, told me I needed to learn some relaxation techniques, stop stressing, see a psychiatrist and get back to life as usual.

I lost it. Not only was I disrespectful to her and frustrated with my family for not understanding my being upset; but I began crying uncontrollably because I had waited for months to see her for some answers. And I was going home with nothing. My hopes had been dashed.

So I went home in full pity party mode and stayed that way for several weeks to come. During my appointment with the neurologist she mentioned something about chronic fatigue but I was so upset that I did not fully absorb what she had said. At some point later when I went to reading again, I came across the words Chronic Fatigue Syndrome.

A few weeks later, I went to see a new general practitioner and she ran a battery of tests and had a fresh outlook and I felt confident that she would get me where I needed to be. In doing her testing, the results were still not conclusive but she did mention Chronic Fatigue Syndrome as well.

So I asked her more about it and what it was and it turns out that Chronic Fatigue Syndrome was also an autoimmune disorder, but does not necessarily affect the right side only. So she was still not convinced. She wanted to investigate the possibility of MS some more, particularly because it ran in my family, on both sides. But after seeing the symptoms associated with Chronic Fatigue and the fact that Candida contributes to that as well, I felt like at least I might have a name for what was ailing me. A name gave me something I could get a cure (or natural remedy) for. So I ran with that. I was tired of feeling bad and wanted to do whatever I could to get my life back.

I started hearing from my friends less once I was no longer the fun spirited girl to hang out or sit and eat at my kitchen table with. People promised to stop in, take me to the store, run errands with and for me, but that only lasted for about two weeks. For everyone else, life went on. My mother was my saving grace and had recently retired. So she devoted several days a week to see that I was cared for and all of my needs were met.

I really started to get angry during this period because I felt as though I had been there for others and they had not shown up for me. And I felt such a deep sense of loneliness. People would call and say, "It's not that serious," and "You'll be alright." But what if I wasn't? How did they know if I would be alright or not? It really began to annoy me that people acted as though I was making it all up and the pain I was feeling was exaggerated.

I later had to come to terms with the fact that everyone else's lives should not stop just because mine had. And further, sometimes people don't have the capacity to give in the same way I do. So I could not hold that against them. I was just bitter because of my circumstances.

One of my girlfriends called me because she'd heard I was dealing with some illness. She, too, had a similar problem some years back and had some mini-strokes but thought she had MS initially. So she understood very clearly what I was dealing with and how I could go from standing up one day to needing a cane the next. Hearing her story was such a help -- to know that I was not exaggerating these aches and pains and that there were many ups and downs with this type of illness. She gave me encouragement and a bit of information that helped me move forward.

A second girlfriend stopped by my place to see me and had no idea my condition had gotten to the point where I truly could not even get around without assistance. She is somewhat of a prophet and she walked to certain places in my home and told me where there was negative energy. And those places were the places where I had been spending most of my time moping about this illness. She prayed with me and gave me a swift kick in the ass and told me to get it together. I took what she said to heart but I still was not quite there yet.

My third visit came from one of my girlfriends who is a breast cancer survivor and one of my high school classmates. She is a true gem and a trooper. She took time out of a busy night of visiting other friends with breast cancer, and later speaking about breast cancer in front of a group of women, to coming by to see about me. She would not take no for an answer. She just needed to lay eyes on me. We talked. We shared. We cried. And once I heard of her battle with cancer, I thought to myself, "How could I even complain about my situation with all that she has been through?" Even though it was still new and challenging for me, she was out praying with others, visiting others, taking people to appointments, conducting speaking engagements and still making time for me...I knew I had to stop feeling sorry for myself. It was serious...but it wasn't that serious. Other people had worse problems than me and did not even complain. My girlfriend ministered to me and told me that the question was not why me but why not me. I am a woman of faith but had allowed this to get the best of me.

It was time to turn the page.

new normal

So I ended the crying spells and decided it was time to take action. My general practitioner said during my last visit, "This might be the best that it is going to be. This might be your new normal. If that is the case, what are you going to do about it? You have to live." So that Sunday after my visit with my girlfriend, I woke up with a plan, decided to take charge of my life and snap back to the old Patrice. That day marked the acceptance of my "new norm". I spent the next several weeks learning about autoimmune diseases and how to heal them. Were there natural remedies or foods that would help heal my body? Are there supplements that will help with the mobility and the pain? If it is MS, what can I do to improve my condition? I could not wait on a diagnosis. Regardless as to what it was, I needed to be proactive. I started coming up with a diet that would balance the reflux, ulcer, Candida, and this unknown disease.

I started researching what supplements would help with muscle spasticity, weakness, tingling and fatigue. I started learning about the benefits of yoga and meditation and the effect stress had on any of the ailments that had been mentioned to me previously.

I started learning that I could do small things but I would now have to pace myself - as one hour-long activity results in up to a week of me being confined to the bed. But at least that was one more hour of activity than I had before.

I began to realize I could not see in the daytime but perhaps I could go out at night. So at least I was not going to be stuck in the house all the time. I just had to be with friends and family that were understanding of my condition and that could get me home or in a comfortable place if an emergency arose.

I began to work on my attitude, which was so important. There are not many days where I don't feel bad, but my days are so much lighter when I don't focus on my illness or my pains.

Going out for me was hard then because I no longer liked the way I looked. With my weight being down, bags under my eyes, blemishes on my skin, I was just not the vibrant person I once was. To make matters worse, I am a fan of high heeled shoes and boots! I only owned three or four pair of flat shoes, outside of tennis shoes and flip flops. So going out was challenging during the winter months because I had no shoes that I could wear that would not cause my energy to plummet or cause me to fall. Wearing heels caused me to be drained almost instantly and were hazardous because I could no longer maintain my balance.

But as I got out more, my confidence grew and I started setting goals for myself. And soon, with enough rest the day before, I was able to drive myself to the grocery store. Then, I was able to walk around the neighborhood for a few minutes. Each week, I tackled a new item on my checklist.

going natural

Even though I felt like I was making strides with my new general practitioner, she even admitted there were some things that she could not help me with as doctors are trained to prescribe medicine for what ails you. If I was unwilling to take medicine, she could only do so much. Considering what I learned about how conventional medicine affects your immune system, and the troubles I had over the years from so many prescription drugs, I refused to take medication unless it was absolutely necessary.

So I began looking up homeopathic doctors and naturopaths in the area. Because I had been eating clean and doing my best to take no western medicines, I thought it might be a good idea to see a naturopath so I could maintain my healthier immune system. Naturopathic medicine is a branch of medicine that focuses on using natural, drug-free therapies to improve overall health. This may include whole food nutrition, herbs, whole food supplements, exercise and other lifestyle modifications. Naturopathic physicians may recommend drug treatments in extreme disease states or emergencies. However, these treatments are usually short-term and only when deemed absolutely necessary.

I settled on the Lifestyle Clinic after doing some research online and speaking to a few naturopathic doctors. I scheduled a consultation with Dr. Kivette Parkes. I immediately connected with her spirit and determined that she would be my doctor. Well, I did not really determine that; but hey, she agreed to take me on as a new patient. During my first visit, she indicated that I had kidney, liver, gall bladder issues and many other things that I never knew I had an issue with just by reading the questionnaire I completed, looking at my skin, and hearing my symptoms. I was impressed! She began treating me for those things but I still was not making much progress. After several months, she had a visiting naturopath sit in on my appointment and review my case.

Based on the large number of symptoms I had they concluded that the only chronic illness that had that many symptoms was Lyme Disease. Due to being a product of the health system for so many years and being as anal as I am, I maintained logs and kept medical records dating back to 1990. But I neglected to inform the doctor that I was bitten by a tick in the early 90s. I did not think that information was relevant at this time. But it turns out that I actually had Lyme Disease for almost 23 years without knowing.

I used to frequent the Sunday afternoon Jazz in the Park during the summer months. One particular Sunday I came home and noticed a rash that covered my entire thigh. I did not immediately seek treatment and used cortisone cream and Benadryl at home. After a week passed and the rash had not disappeared, and along with it came a fever and chills, I then went to the doctor and was told I had been bitten by a tick. I was never informed that there could be serious consequences down the road; only that I may suffer from some minor muscle aches and pains over the next year or two, due to the amount of time that had passed before I sought a doctor's care.

the great imitator

Lyme Disease is an infectious disease caused by the bacteria Borrelia burgdorferi. In the early stages, 4-8 weeks immediately following infection, the disease can most often be successfully eradicated by aggressive antibiotic treatment. There are three stages to Lyme Disease:

Stage 1: Early Localized Lyme Disease - Early infection occurs in one to four weeks where individuals may feel flu like symptoms and exhibit fever, sore and tired muscles, headache and fatigue. Some will develop the bullseye rash, but not all.

Stage 2: Early Disseminated Lyme Disease - Occurs several weeks after the tick bite. Individuals may exhibit swollen lymph nodes, vision changes, pain and weakness, muscle aches, and have a general feeling of malaise. Some experience Bell's Palsy and many neurological symptoms in this stage.

Stage 3: Late Disseminated, Late Stage or Chronic Lyme Disease - Can occur, weeks, months or even years after the tick bite. Occurs when the infection was not properly treated in Stages 1 or 2. In this stage, the Lyme affects the neurological and nervous system and many other organs. Individuals may experience severe headache pain, arthritis and joint pain and stiffness, heart disturbances, insomnia, circulatory issues, digestive issues, skin issues, memory loss, difficulty concentrating and mental fogginess, fatigue, numbness and muscle weakness.

Lyme disease becomes chronic when the bacteria moves inside the body tissues and cells and starts affecting different body systems. Chronic Lyme is much more difficult to address since it is not possible to destroy the bacteria once it is inside the cells. Antibiotic treatment can keep the bacteria from spreading, but the long term effects of prolonged antibiotic use can be devastating for some patients. Additionally, ticks may carry several other diseases so a patient may also have co-infections, which often make diagnosing and treating Lyme more difficult.

People affected with Lyme disease are often treated by various medical specialists for years without being properly diagnosed because the symptoms can change rapidly. Many patients choose to pursue a

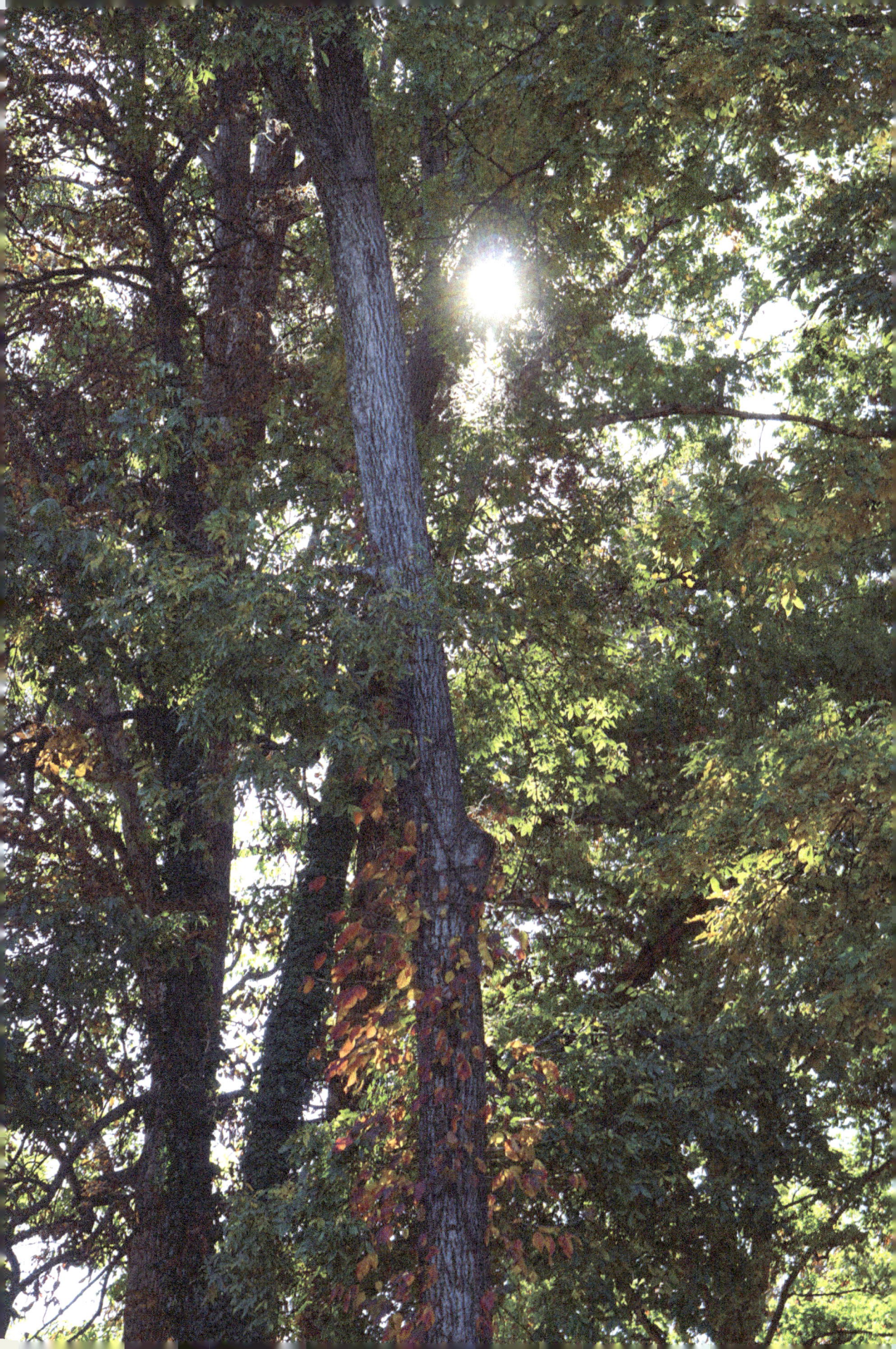

naturopathic approach because those physicians focus on the root cause of the disease, which is a derangement in the immune system. This approach addresses the underlying cause of the symptoms and allows patients to rebuild their bodies and improve their overall health long term. Lyme Disease is notoriously known as the Great Imitator and can mimic over 300 diseases. Since the underlying effects of Chronic Lyme disease is a significantly overburdened immune system, people with the disease are often plagued with a variety of other infections that are difficult to handle - infections caused by viruses, yeast, bacteria, fungi and even parasites. Since these pathogens are opportunistic, it is easier for them to replicate and infect a person with Chronic Lyme disease because their immune system is unable to protect them.

Initially, I made a lifestyle change because I wanted to stop taking western medicines and cut back on antibiotic use. Now, with Late Stage Lyme Disease (Stage 3) it was imperative that I maintain a clean eating diet. The most significant burden placed on the immune system is one in which we have complete control over - our food.

The immune system reacts directly to food. So if the body is constantly inundated with foods that trigger inflammation or allergic reactions, the immune system is overburdened and symptoms of Lyme (or any chronic illness) worsen. When managing or preventing disease, or just trying to live a healthier lifestyle, one should adapt to a whole food, vegetable based diet with chemical free meats and foods.

One of the reasons I struggled with illness was because of the havoc I wreaked on my body that was tearing down my immune system and causing inflammation - eating the wrong foods, not getting proper rest, and consuming foods with gluten in them. So I later removed yeast, gluten and pork from my diet as well. I will eat red meat on rare occasions but not very often, as it causes issues for my digestive system.

So while I am forced to eat this way to maintain a healthier lifestyle, this cookbook is not just for people who suffer from Lyme Disease or any chronic illness. I wrote this book to illustrate that clean eating and natural remedies are not bland, they do work, and foods are actually all you need to heal most of what ails the body. I am not a trained chef or a medical professional; just someone who has a passion for food and healthy living. With my new lifestyle, I can count on one hand the number of times I have had to take conventional medicine since I started this process in 2010. I have cured many of my colds, sinus infections, flu bugs, rashes, sore throat pain, ear infections, allergies, constipation and bloating all through healing foods, natural supplements and medicines and the use of essential oils. And so can you!

All of these recipes are free of gluten, sugar, yeast and little to no dairy. And all of my meat selections are grass fed or antibiotic free. So, strengthen your immunity, boost your vitality and start your journey towards a healthier lifestyle today!

dried oregano

coriander

dried rosemary

sage

black pepper

thyme

smoked paprika

cinnamon

turmeric

cumin

himalayan pink salt

spices in my kitchen
that are good for your health too!

Oregano
Oregano is not just good for your pizza sauces and Mediterranean dishes! I deal with a lot of pain and muscle aches with Lyme Disease. I use dried oregano in an herbal tea, for muscle aches, nausea and bloating. You can find oregano oil in most health food stores and it is great for bacterial, viral and fungal infections.

Coriander
Coriander is known to help with issues of anemia and eye health. Coriander is also great for digestion. Pair it with cumin and fennel for a calming tea that reduces bloating and gas.

Rosemary
I love using rosemary in healthy drinks or cocktails, for you non-clean eating folks! It is also great for boosting circulation, boosting the immune system and detoxifying the body. Rosemary essential oil is also great for some forms of hair loss and is great for relieving congestion.

Black Pepper
There is something about cracked black pepper which is a little more robust than pre-ground pepper. With whole peppercorns, the flavor is locked inside so it is much more flavorful. But I also add black pepper to my warm turmeric drinks, as it helps provide maximum absorption when paired together.

Thyme
Thyme is a great herb for cooking in breads, roasted vegetables, poultry dishes and sauces; but it is great for alleviating sinus and bronchitis issues as well.

Sage
Sage is used for digestive problems, loss of appetite, gas, diarrhea, bloating, and heartburn. Because I suffer from a lot of kidney and liver issues, I steep the leaves to make a tea with it as well. When not using it for medicinal purposes, I will often have it in my poultry dishes.

Smoked Paprika
Move over paprika! Smoked paprika is my new favorite spice. I love to use it in marinades, on corn on the cob, deviled eggs, and to season my boneless, skinless chicken breasts. While not as pungent as cayenne pepper, it does have a nice, smoky flavor. The capsaicin found in paprika has anti-inflammatory properties, which can ease joint pain.

Cinnamon
I use cinnamon a good bit. In teas, in savory dishes, in pies and sweet dishes. Cinnamon has impressive health benefits to include anti-inflammatory properties, it fights viruses and infections, and helps with allergies.

Turmeric
I use turmeric mainly for Indian dishes, soups and curries. But turmeric is great for pain relief and is an anti-inflammatory. Use it in teas and smoothies for a nutritional boost.

Himalayan Pink Salt
I commonly use Kosher salt, but also cook with Himalayan pink salt, which is known for its high nutritional content. I also use Himalayan pink salt in my detox baths to release toxins.

Cumin
Cumin is a savory, nutty spice with a distinctive taste that I use in stews, Indian dishes, savory dishes, soups, sweet potatoes and teas. Cumin is said to aid in digestion, improve immunity and treat hemorrhoids, insomnia, and respiratory issues.

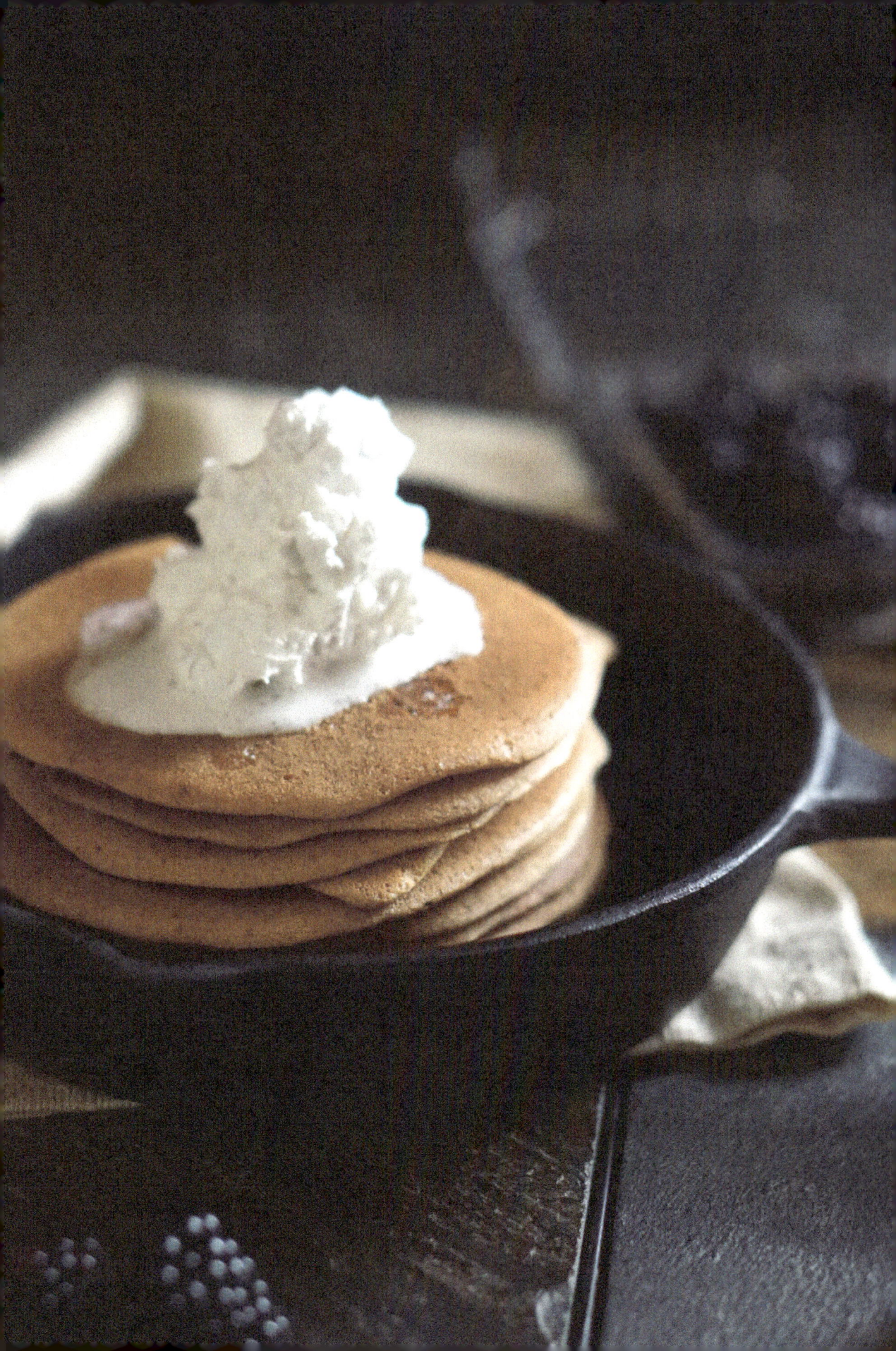

breakfast

24 Quinoa Porridge
Get your amino acids and proteins all in one breakfast bowl.

26 Fried Egg 'n Hash
Luscious fried egg with a hash of chicken apple sausage, Brussels sprouts, sweet potatoes and apples.

28 Blueberry Muffins
Simple, delicious breakfast that tastes as good as the non gluten-free variety.

29 Homemade Granola
No need to buy granola in the store when it is so easy to make at home.

32 Parfait
Turn that homemade granola into an amazing breakfast parfait.

34 Brown Rice Pancakes
Take your leftover brown rice to use in this hearty pancake dish.

36 Gluten Free Pancakes
Something about pancakes and Saturday mornings...

37 Frittata
A hearty frittata, good for breakfast or dinner, that looks like it took hours to make.

40 Kale Smoothie
Get your greens in with this high-fiber smoothie.

41 Antioxidant Smoothie
Get an antioxidant boost with this quick, but potent, smoothie.

42 Avocado Smoothie
This creamy smoothie is a great meal replacement for breakfast on the run.

44 Apple Pie Smoothie
This smoothie is filling, savory and tastes like apple pie in a glass.

46 Sweet Potato Smoothie
Get a punch of essential nutrients with this healthy breakfast smoothie.

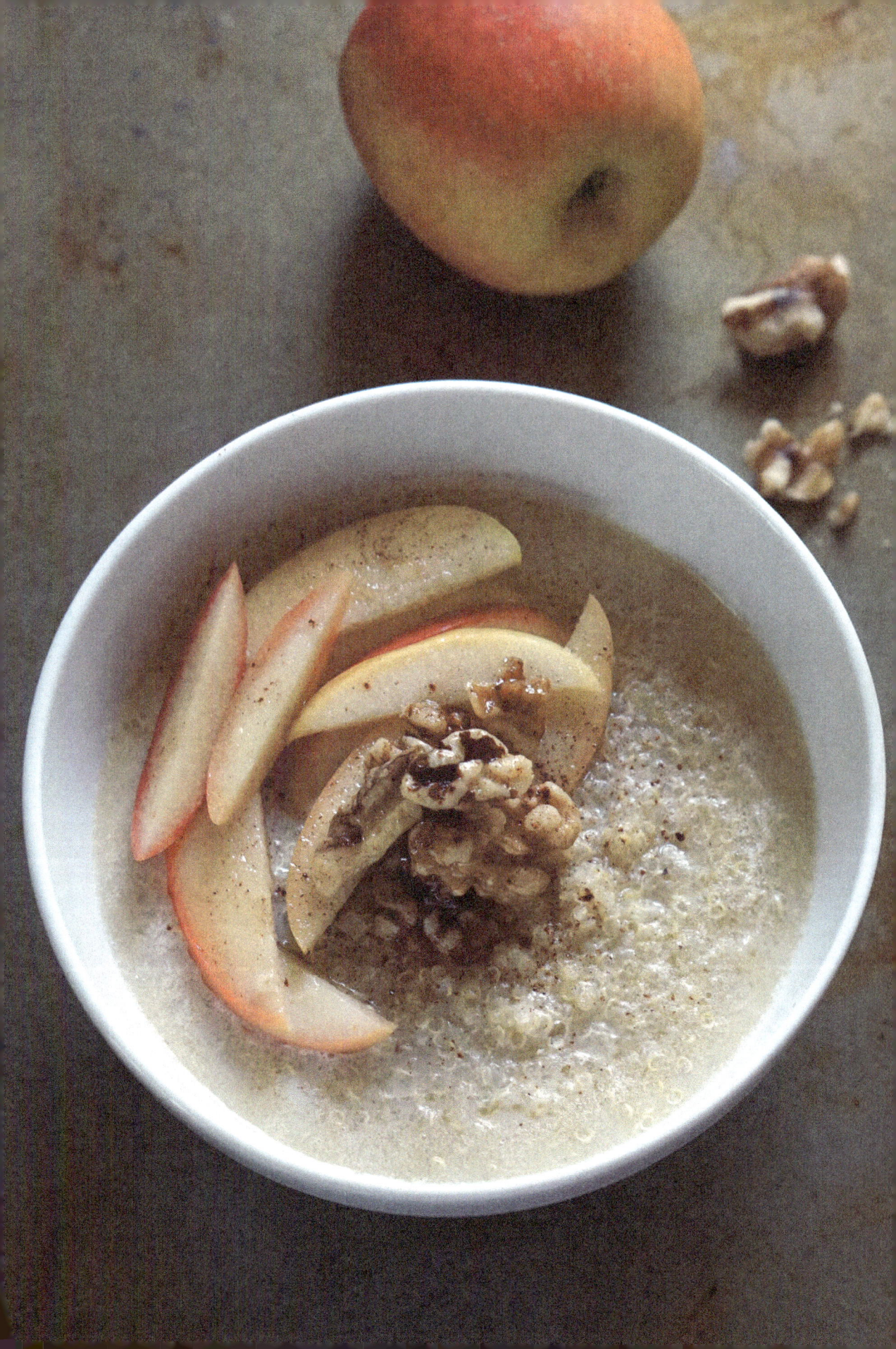

quinoa porridge

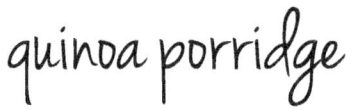

[Serves 2]

Quinoa is an acquired taste for many. And it can definitely be unappealing if you do not rinse it properly before using it in your favorite dish. But if you enjoy it, this porridge is a nutritious alternative to oatmeal or my beloved Cream of Wheat. Quinoa is naturally gluten-free and is considered a complete protein, containing all of the essential amino acids. Get some!

1 cup cooked quinoa
1 tablespoon butter
2 cups water

1 - 1 1/2 cup almond milk
2 teaspoons stevia

Optional:
Sprinkle of ground cinnamon and nutmeg
1 teaspoon ground flax seeds
Fruit compote or fresh fruit
Toasted nuts

Rinse quinoa for about 5 minutes (or until the water runs clear) to get rid of saponin.

Place cup quinoa, 1 tablespoon butter and 2 cups water in a saucepan and bring to a boil. Reduce to a simmer, cover and cook until all water is absorbed, 10-15 minutes.

Once all of the water is absorbed, pour almond milk over quinoa and heat just slightly, until the milk is warmed.

Pour into a bowl, add stevia or raw honey (to taste), sprinkle with spices and with flax seeds or fruit and nuts, if you desire.

.....
Be sure to rinse your quinoa thoroughly before cooking so that the bitter taste from the saponin is not present.

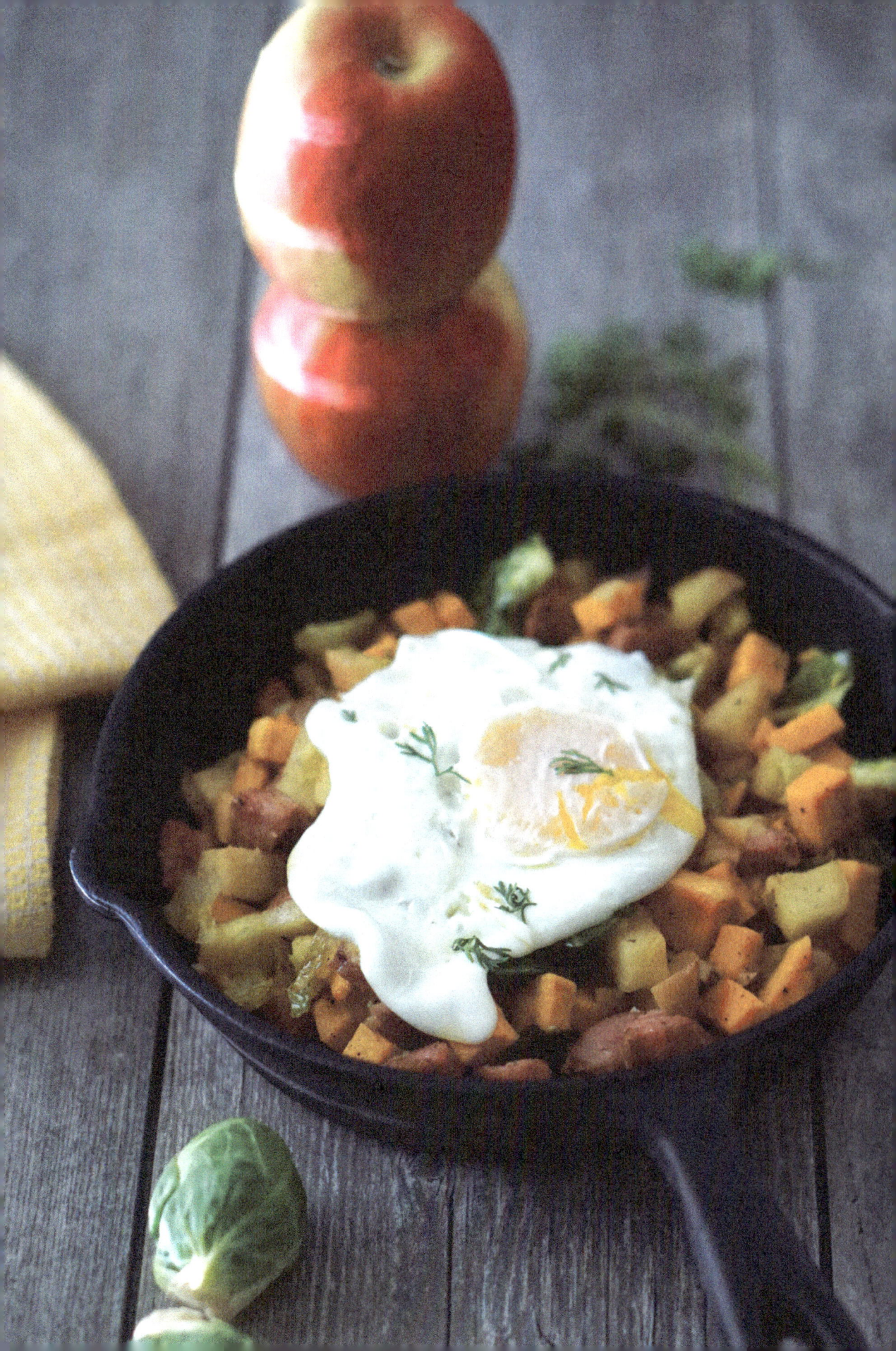

fried egg 'n hash

[Serves 2]

When I did my first major detox and could not have eggs for a month, I got real creative with breakfast. I was alternating between stir fry and this hash, which is pretty amazing by itself, but even better with a fried egg on top. For those who are used to pancakes, bacon and eggs, or your more traditional breakfast dishes, maybe it is time to switch it up a bit! This recipe uses some of my favorite produce...it's a very hearty, savory dish.

1 medium sweet potato, peeled and cubed
2 cups Brussels sprouts, quartered
2 tablespoons coconut or olive oil, divided
2 chicken apple sausages, chopped
2 Rome or Gala apples, cubed
1 medium yellow onion, chopped
2 cloves garlic, minced
Kosher salt and ground black pepper to taste
1/2 teaspoon cumin
1/2 teaspoon nutmeg
1/2 cup chicken stock

Bring a medium stock pot of water to a boil. Add sweet potato cubes and Brussels sprouts and cook for 5-7 minutes, until sweet potatoes are almost tender. Remove from heat and drain. Set aside.

Heat 1 tablespoon of the oil in a large, nonstick skillet over medium high heat. Add the chicken apple sausage and cook for approximately 5 minutes.

Reduce heat and add Brussels sprouts, sweet potato cubes, apples and yellow onion. Cook, stirring occasionally, until the onions are translucent, about 5-8 minutes.

Add the garlic, and seasonings. Cook for 5 minutes and then add chicken stock. Cook for another 3-5 minutes and serve.

Optional: Top with a fried or poached egg.

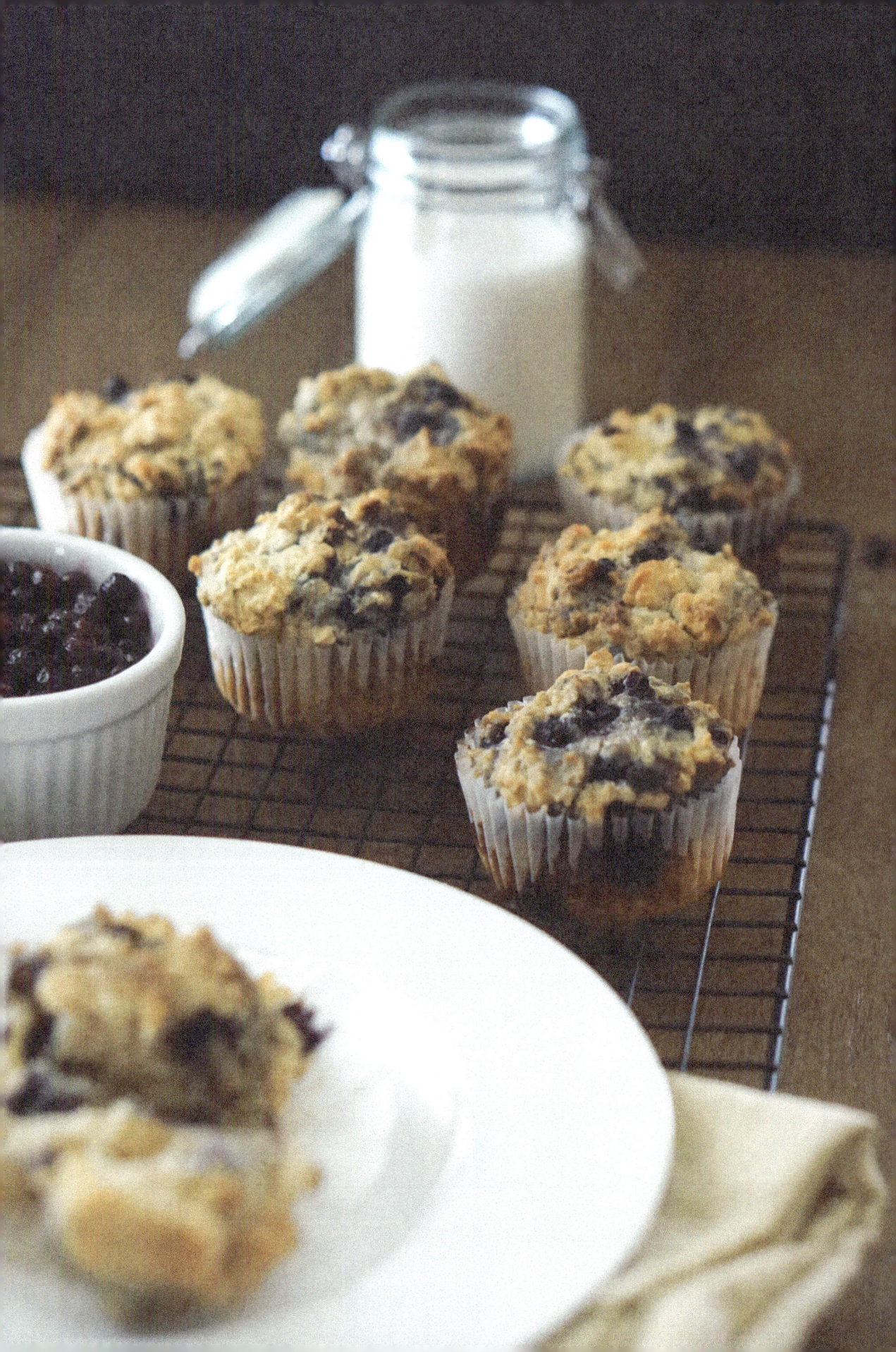

blueberry muffins

[Serves 4]

I have fond memories of Saturday mornings as a youngin' when Mominski made scrambled eggs and those boxed blueberry muffins. I don't love blueberries on their own; but love them in muffins and smoothies. And these muffins are so tasty you would almost not know they were gluten-free and good for you! Sprinkle the top with stevia and walnuts before baking if you want a nice, crispy topping.

1 1/4 cup gluten free flour blend
2 teaspoons baking powder
1/2 teaspoon sea salt
1/2 cup stevia in the raw
1 large egg
1 cup almond milk
1/3 cup coconut oil, melted
1 cup frozen organic blueberries
Lemon zest

Preheat the oven to 350 degrees. Line a standard 12-cup muffin tin with paper liners.

In a medium bowl, whisk together the flour, baking powder, salt and stevia.

In a mixing bowl, blend the egg, milk, and melted coconut oil together.

Add the dry ingredients to the wet ingredients and mix until the batter is smooth. Using a spatula, gently fold in the blueberries and lemon zest just until they are evenly distributed throughout the batter.

Fill the muffin cups until almost full. Bake the muffins for 25-30 minutes or until a toothpick comes out clean when inserted in the center.

Let muffins stand for 10 minutes before transferring them to a wire rack to cool completely.

.....

To keep your blueberries from sinking, toss them in a teaspoon of flour to lightly coat them and gently fold them in as the very last step before putting the batter in the muffin pan.

homemade granola

[Serves 2]

This homemade granola is so easy and can be customized to fit whatever suits you. You can change up the nuts/seeds, add dried fruits...make it your own! Preparing it at home also allows you to control how much sugar is incorporated, which is a huge benefit from purchasing store-bought granola.

2 cups gluten free oats
½ cup raw nuts (almonds, walnuts), chopped
¼ cup shredded unsweetened coconut
¼ cup raw seeds (pumpkin, sesame seeds)
½ cup unsweetened dried fruit, *optional*
3 tablespoons virgin coconut oil, melted
A pinch of sea salt
1 dropper of liquid stevia or
2 tablespoons raw honey

Preheat oven to 250 degrees.

Combine all ingredients in a large mixing bowl. Spread the mixture in thin layer on a baking sheet and bake for 60-75 minutes, stirring halfway through the baking process to achieve even color.

Cool completely and store in an airtight container.

.....
Bake your granola at a lower temperature and continue to stir the mixture to ensure it does not burn - and that it browns evenly.

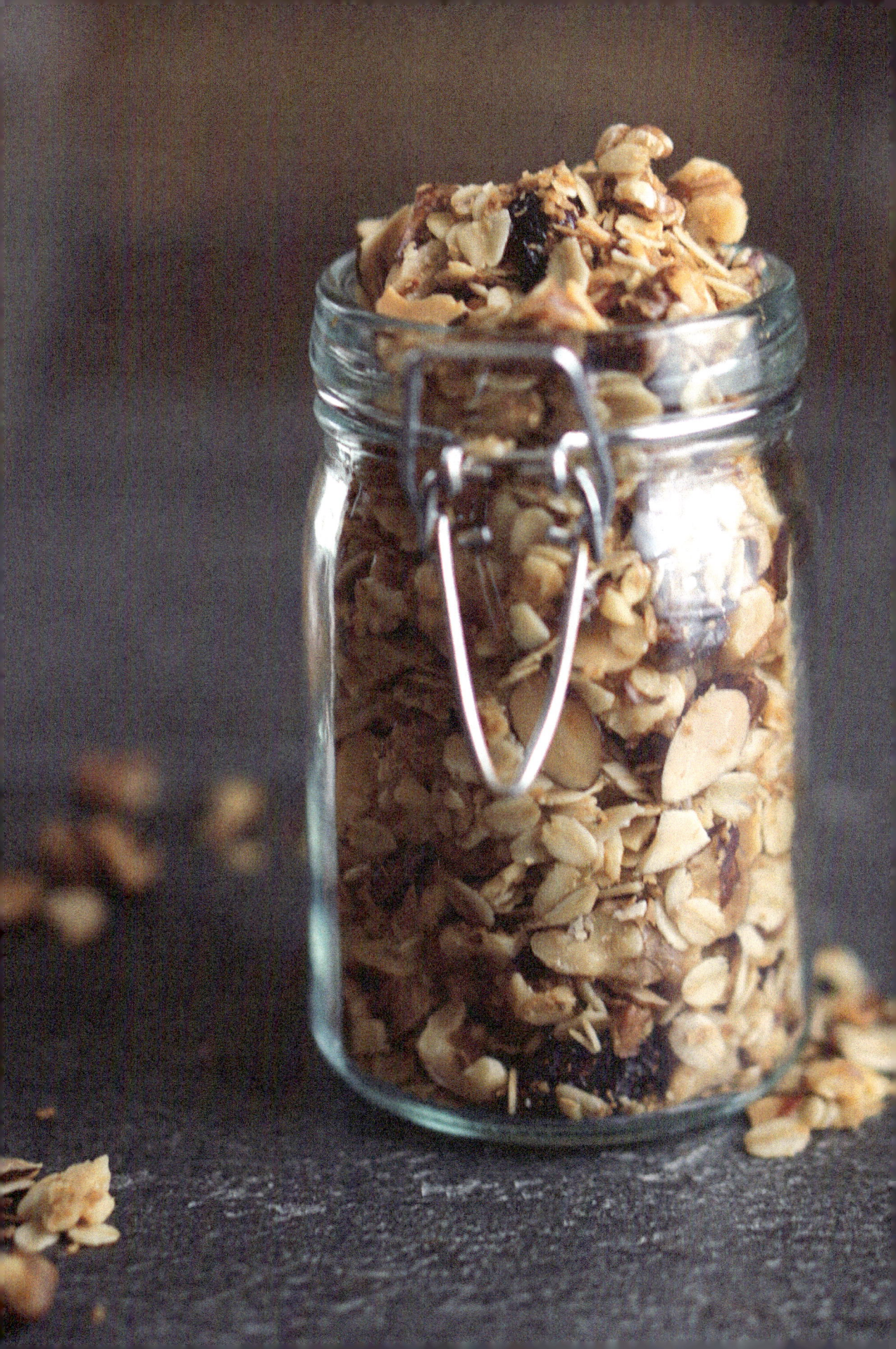

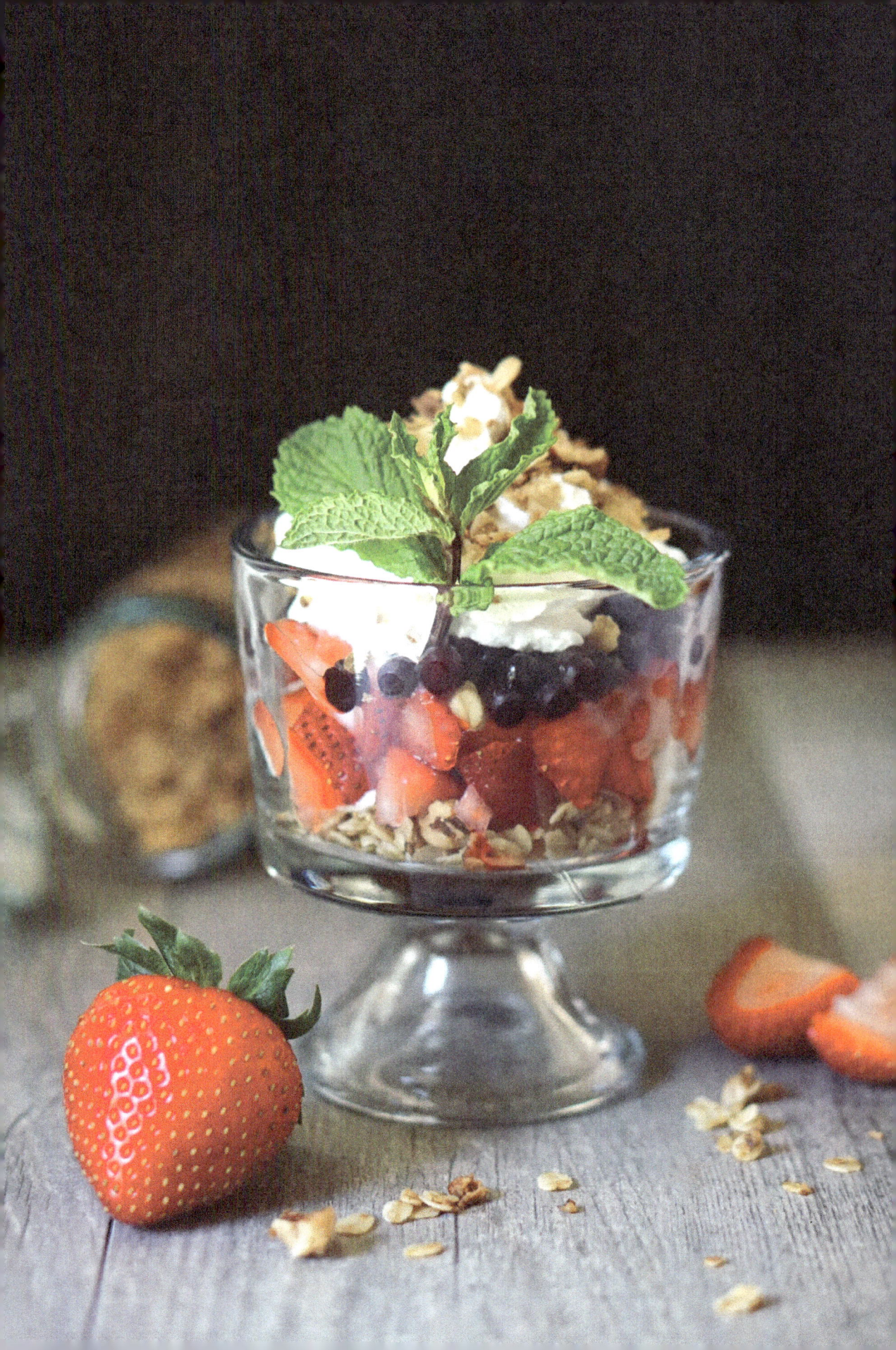

parfait

[Serves 2]

I am eternally grateful to whomever created coconut cream...and full fat coconut milk! I am never without it and the both can be used in so many different ways. In baked goods, ice cream, as mayonnaise, sour cream and as a whipped topping. This quick and easy parfait is perfect for breakfast (or dessert) and is aesthetically pleasing for a Memorial Day or Fourth of July cookout or celebration!

1 can coconut cream
Liquid stevia, to taste
2 cups of fresh strawberries
1/2 cup of fresh raspberries
1/2 cup of fresh blueberries
1 cup Homemade Granola

Whipped Coconut Cream:

Refrigerate the can of coconut cream overnight. (I prefer Trader Joe's version of coconut cream). Chill your beaters in the freezer, along with the mixing bowl, for a minimum of 15 minutes.

Scrape the coconut cream from the can, tossing the liquid. Place the coconut cream in the chilled mixing bowl and whip until thick and creamy. Add liquid stevia and whip for a minute longer to incorporate the sweetener. Adjust if needed. Place in refrigerator until ready to assemble parfait.

Homemade Granola:

[See recipe on page 27]

Assemble Parfait:

Layer ingredients in a glass - add berries, cream, then granola and repeat until glass is full. Top with cream and a sprinkle of granola. Serve!

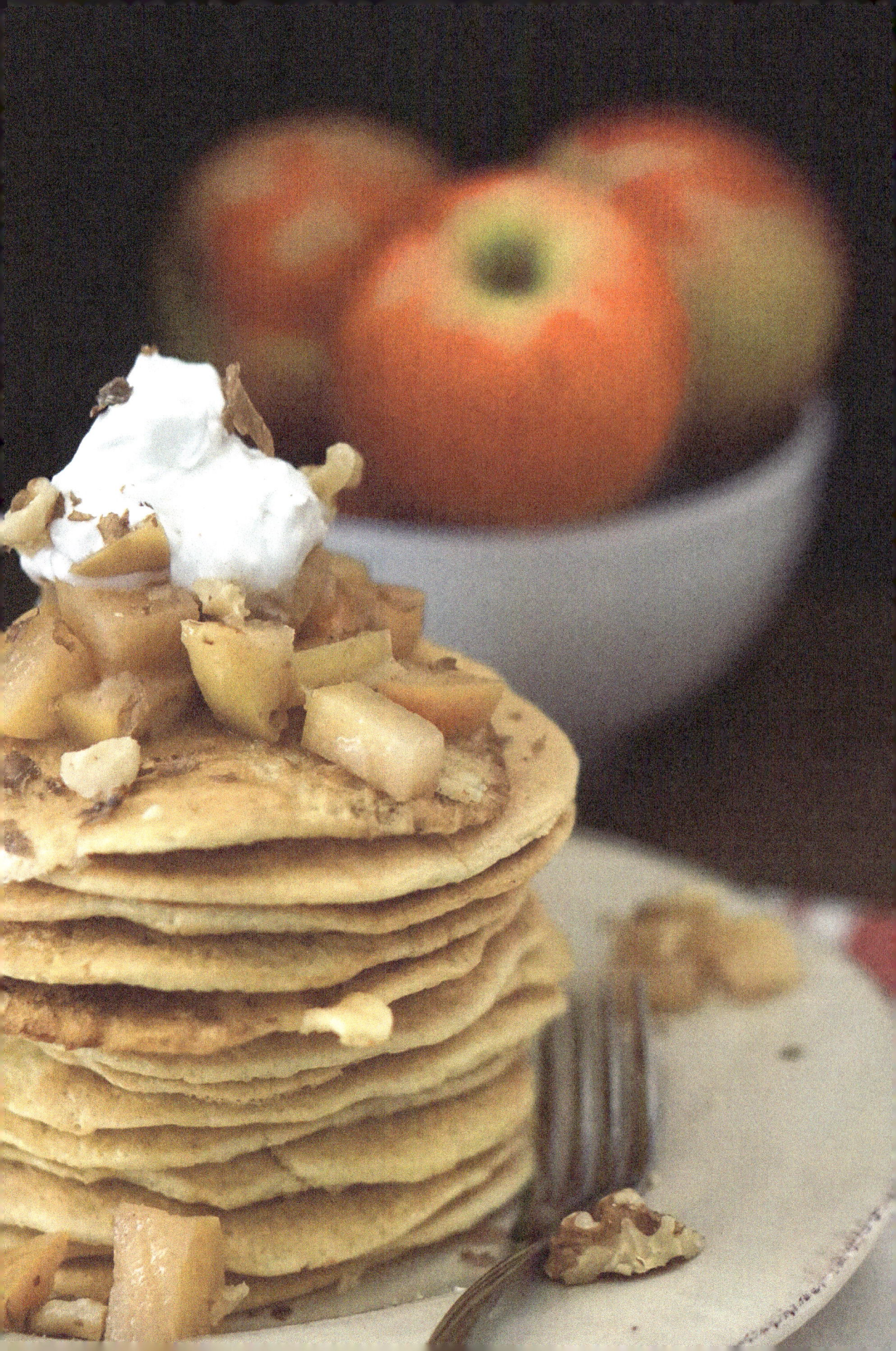

brown rice pancakes

[Serves 2]

Pancakes were my weekend thing. Before I ran my errands or even got out of my pj's, I would make my hot tea, my turkey bacon and my pancake stack. If you want to enjoy them during the week and are pressed for time, make the batter a day ahead and store it in the fridge overnight. These pancakes are a great way to use leftover brown rice.

4 organic eggs, separated
1 cup cooked brown rice
1 cup almond milk, unsweetened
1/2 teaspoon salt
2 tablespoons stevia
6 tablespoons brown rice flour
2 tablespoons butter

Beat egg yolks. Incorporate cooked rice, milk, salt, stevia, flour, cinnamon and butter and blend well.

In a large bowl beat egg whites until stiff peaks form. Gently fold into batter.

Heat butter on a griddle or in cast iron pan. Cook pancakes until bubbles form. Flip on other side and cook for another minute or until done.

gluten free pancakes

[Serves 2-3]

For these pancakes, I tend to like the combination of an all purpose gluten free flour and a whole grain gluten free flour, but you can use a brown rice and a gluten-free blend as well or just gluten free flour, though they may not be quite as rich. Top with a fruit compote, almond butter, honey, nuts, or...you guessed it...coconut cream!

1 3/4 cups unsweetened almond milk
1 tablespoon organic apple cider vinegar
1 cup gluten free all purpose flour
1 cup gluten free whole grain flour
1/4 cup stevia
2 teaspoons baking powder
1 teaspoon baking soda
1 teaspoon salt
2 eggs, beaten
2 tablespoons butter, melted

Add organic apple cider vinegar to the almond milk and let stand for 10 minutes to sour.

In a bowl, combine flours and remaining dry ingredients. In a separate bowl, combine the wet ingredients. Combine the wet and dry ingredients and mix just until blended.

Heat a griddle or in cast iron pan. Do not add additional butter or oil to cook with if using a griddle. Cook pancakes until bubbles form. Flip on other side and cook for another minute or until done.

Note: For the flours, I enjoy using King Arthur Flour's Gluten-Free Whole Grain Flour Blend and Trader Joe's Gluten Free All Purpose Flour.

.....
Gluten free pancakes are typically much flatter than pancakes made with regular flour. If you want to add a bit of fluff to your pancakes, beat the egg whites until stiff peaks form and gently fold them into the pancake batter.

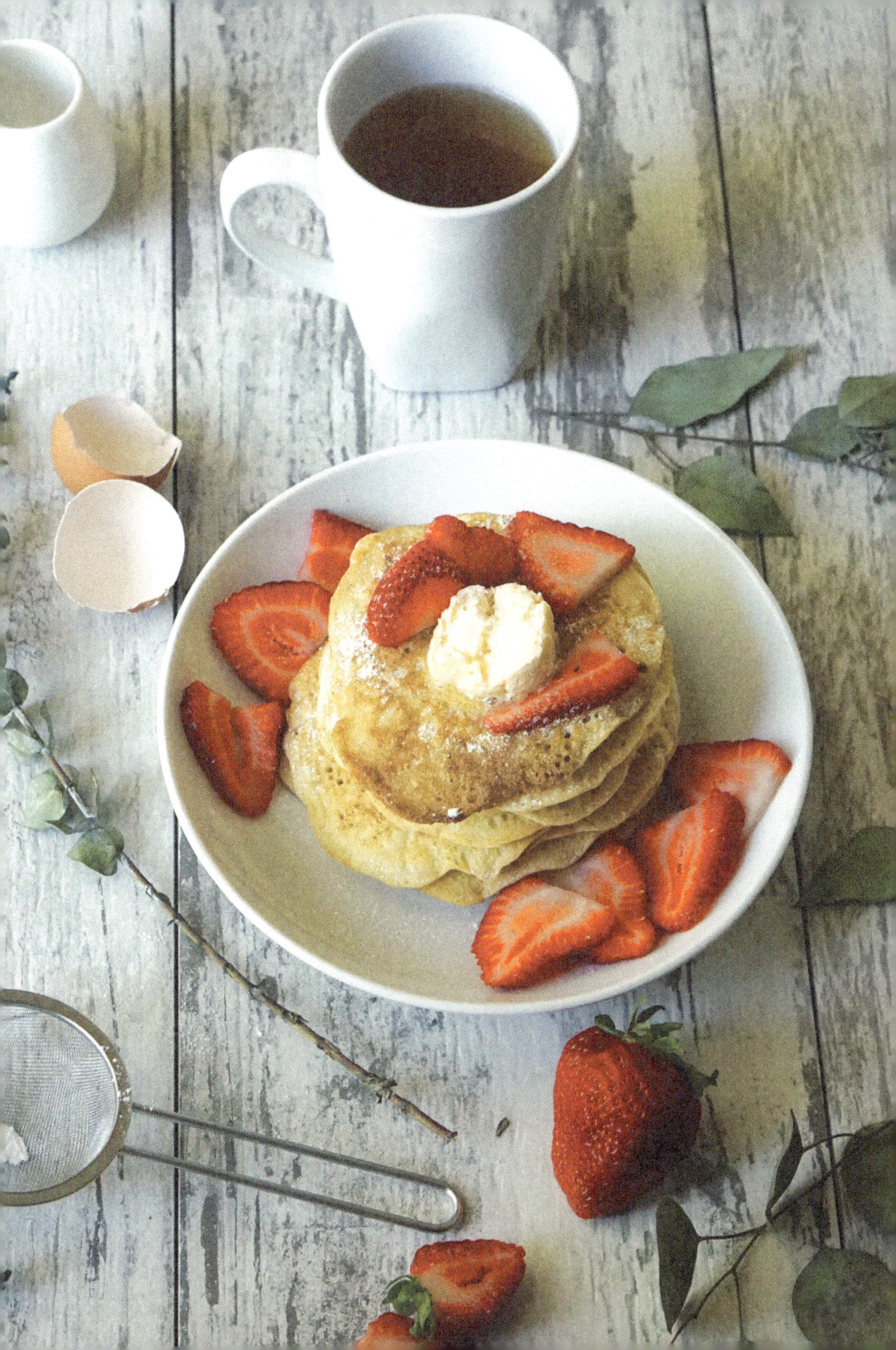

kale and goat cheese frittata

[Serves 4]

This is such a beautiful dish and looks like it took hours to prepare. This frittata is great for breakfast or a weeknight dinner, along with an arugula or kale salad or a bowl of fresh fruit.

1 tablespoon olive oil
1 small red onion, diced
2 handfuls of chopped curly kale
1/2 cup shiitake mushrooms
1 cup grape tomatoes, sliced
8 large farm fresh eggs, lightly beaten
Salt and freshly ground black pepper
Goat cheese or cheese alternative, such as Vegan Gourmet or Daiya

Heat oven to 375 degrees.

Heat the olive oil in a cast iron pan. Add the onions and cook until translucent. Add the kale, mushrooms and tomatoes and cook for 5 minutes until the kale has wilted.

Lightly beat the eggs. Season with salt and pepper. Add the eggs to the cast iron pan, evenly distributing the mixture. Cook on low heat for 5 minutes, until the egg is nearly set.

Scatter the cheese over the top of the frittata. Cook in the oven for approximately 15-18 minutes, until the frittata is completely set in the center.

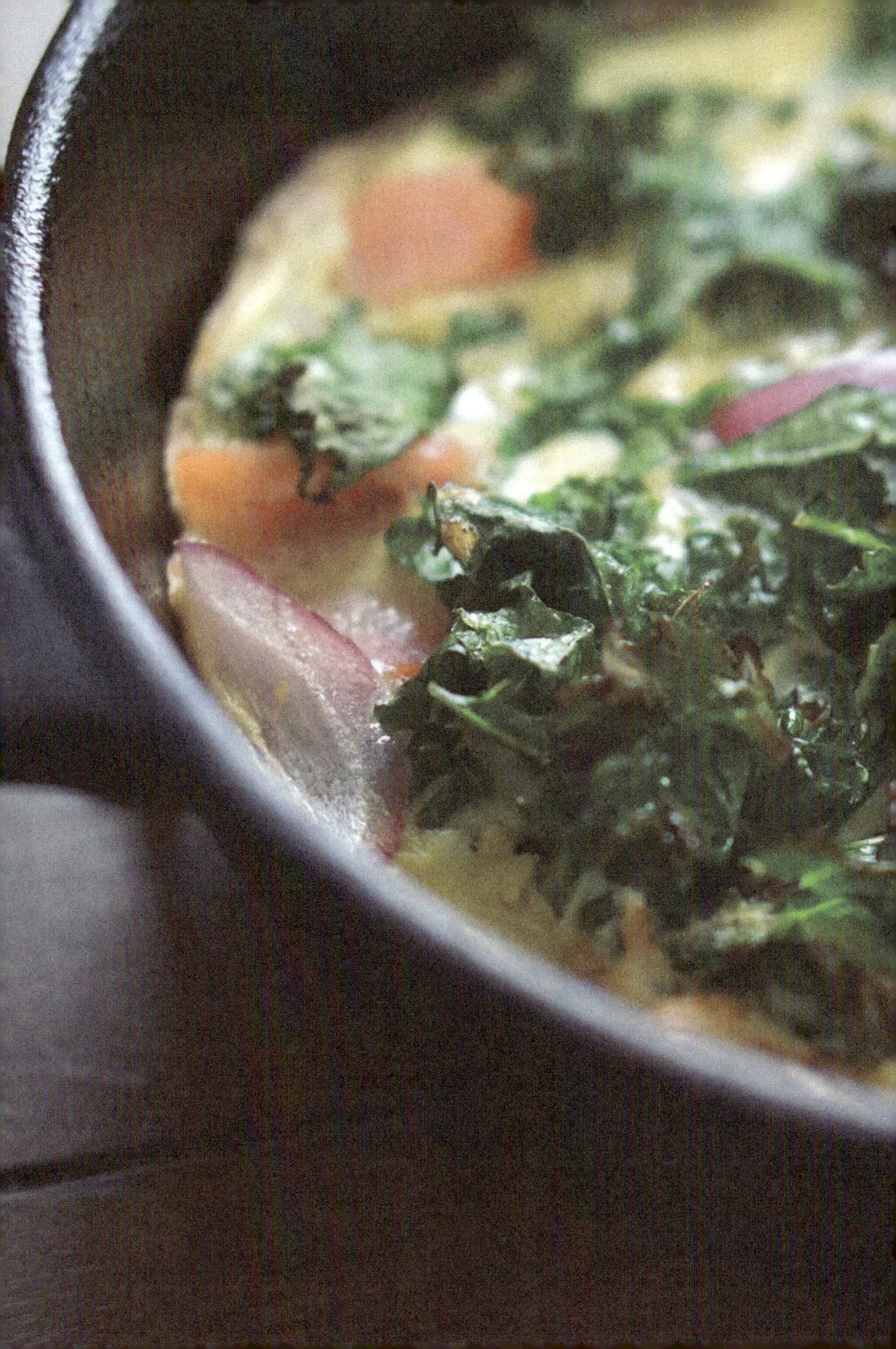

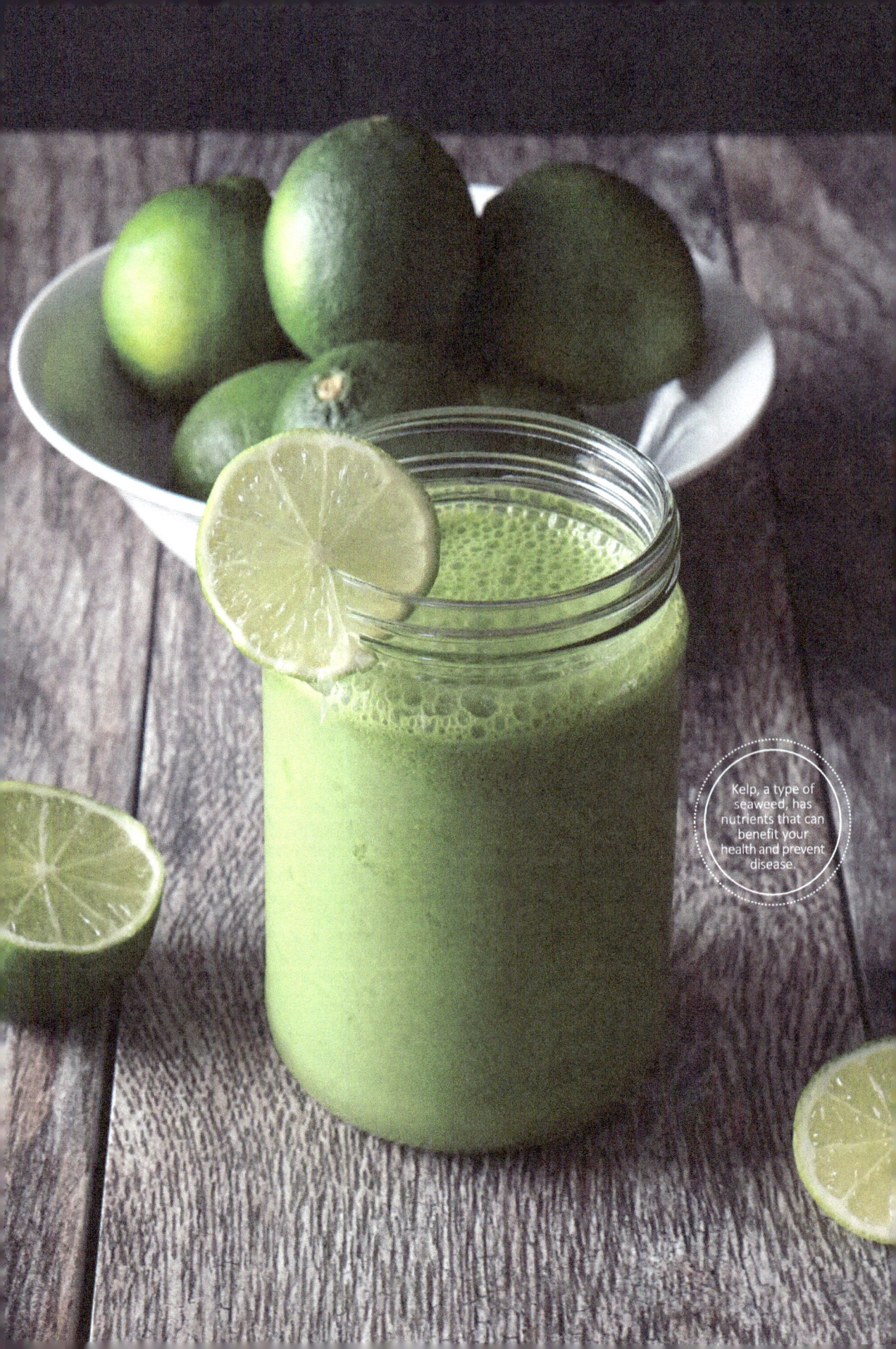

Kelp, a type of seaweed, has nutrients that can benefit your health and prevent disease.

kale smoothie

[Serves 1]

A lot of people are intimidated by green smoothies because of their color and high vegetable content; but if you add a little fruit to your green smoothies, you will hardly notice the vegetables are even in there. Kale is high in fiber so it is great for aiding in digestion. It also gives you an energy boost and is how I keep my clear skin! Drink up!

16 oz. almond/coconut blend milk
2 scoops vanilla protein powder
1 teaspoon almond butter, *optional*
Handful of kale
1 small Golden Delicious apple
1 teaspoon stevia
1 handful of ice

Variation:
12 oz. almond milk
Juice of one small lime
Handful of kale
1 teaspoon flaxseed oil
1/2 avocado
1 teaspoon stevia
1 handful of ice

Process ingredients in blender until smooth. Serve.

.....
You can use any kind of kale for smoothies but be warned that lacinato kale is going to be very bitter.

antioxidant smoothie

[Serves 1]

Antioxidants help prevent or stop cell damage caused by harmful molecules. The benefits of antioxidants are essential to good health because if free radicals are left unchallenged, they can cause a wide range of illnesses. Enjoy the benefits and goodness of this fruity smoothie along with your next breakfast.

4 oz. water	Process ingredients in blender until smooth. Serve.
4 oz. unsweetened cranberry juice	
1/2 cup frozen blueberries	
1/2 cup frozen strawberries	
1 teaspoon coconut oil	
1 teaspoon stevia	
1 handful of ice	

.....
If you don't have flaxseed oil on hand, substitute ground flaxseed, which is easier to find in the grocery stores.

avocado smoothie

[Serves 1]

One of the things that I try to incorporate in my day-to-day routine is drinking a fresh juice or smoothie. Smoothies and fresh juices are a great way to get your recommended fruits and veggies in a quick and easy manner. Avocado smoothies are a great meal replacement drink as they can be very filling. Packed with healthy fats, this is a nutritious way to start the day.

16 oz. almond milk
1/2 avocado
2 scoops vanilla protein powder
1 small green apple
1 handful spinach
1 kelp tablet, *optional*
1 teaspoon stevia
1 handful of ice

Variation:
12 oz. coconut milk
1/2 avocado
Juice of one small lime
1 handful spinach
1/2 cup honeydew
1 teaspoon spirulina
1 teaspoon stevia
1 handful of ice

Process ingredients in blender until smooth. Serve.

.....

If you do not like the taste of stevia, you can substitute raw honey for sweetness. Stay away from agave, and those little pink, blue and yellow packets.

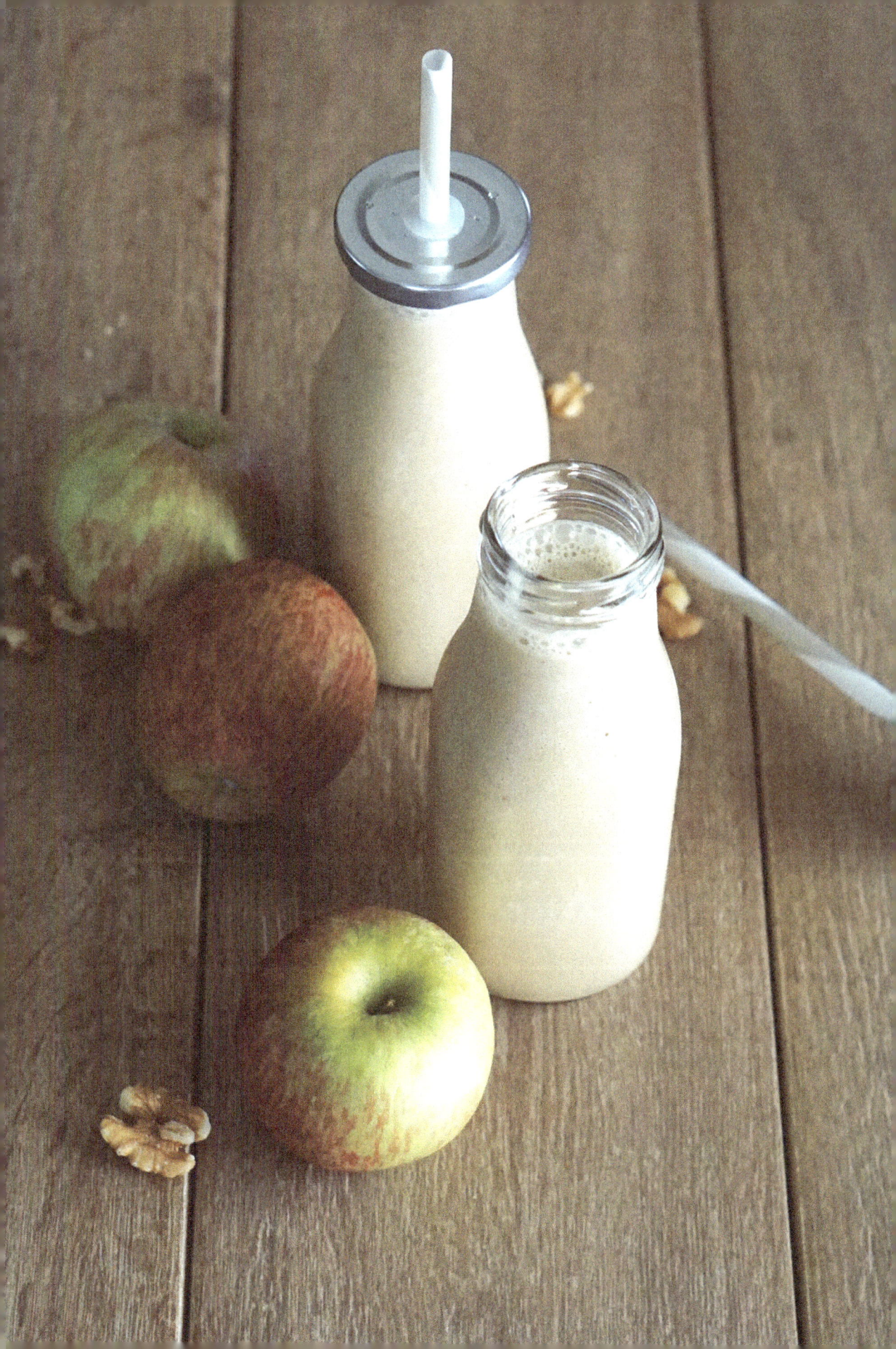

apple pie smoothie

[Serves 1]

Don't get bogged down with the traditional fruit smoothies made with berries, mangoes and bananas. This smoothie is a good meal replacement smoothie and is like having oatmeal or apple pie in a glass! Because this does not contain any frozen fruit, it will not be as thick as a typical smoothie but if you like a thicker consistency, add a bit of coconut cream or more rolled oats and ice to the mixture.

12 oz. almond milk
1 small red apple, cored
2 scoops vanilla protein powder
1/4 cup rolled oats, uncooked
1 teaspoon almond butter
Dash of cinnamon
Dash of nutmeg
Dash of turmeric
1 teaspoon flaxseed
1 teaspoon stevia
1 handful of ice

Process ingredients in blender until smooth. Serve.

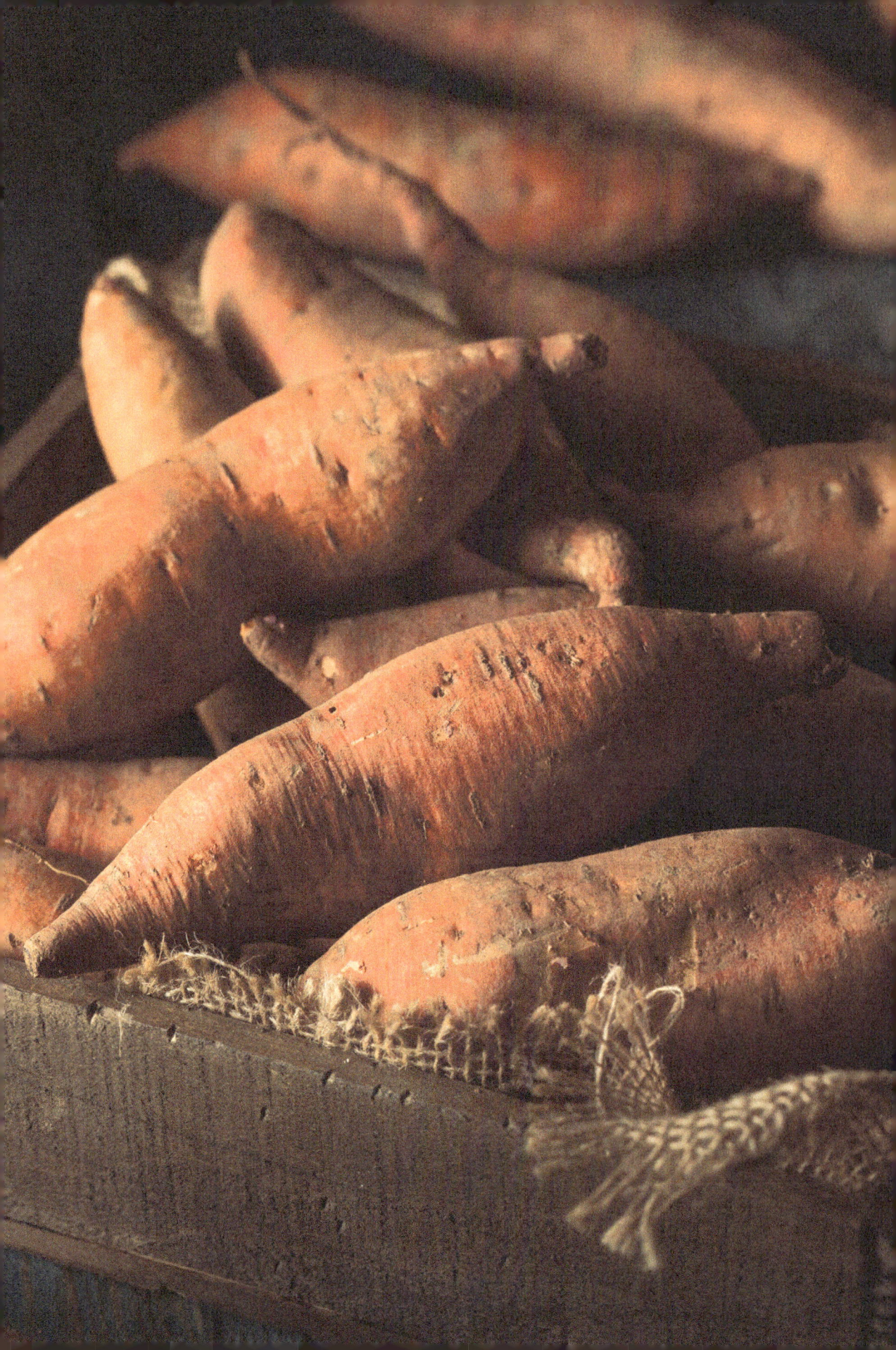

sweet potato smoothie

[Serves 1]

This smoothie reminds me of fall, comfort food and sweet potato pie. You may want to adjust the amount of stevia based on the ripeness of your banana. If you are on a low (natural) sugar diet, you can eliminate the banana altogether and it will be just as pleasing.

16 oz. coconut (or almond) milk
1/4 cup freshly squeezed orange juice
1/2 cup cooked sweet potato
1/2 of frozen banana
Dash of cinnamon powder
Dash of ginger powder
Dash of turmeric
1 teaspoon stevia
1 handful of ice

Process ingredients in blender until smooth. Serve.

.....
Add a little turmeric powder to this drink to give you a boost! Turmeric is a great anti-inflammatory.

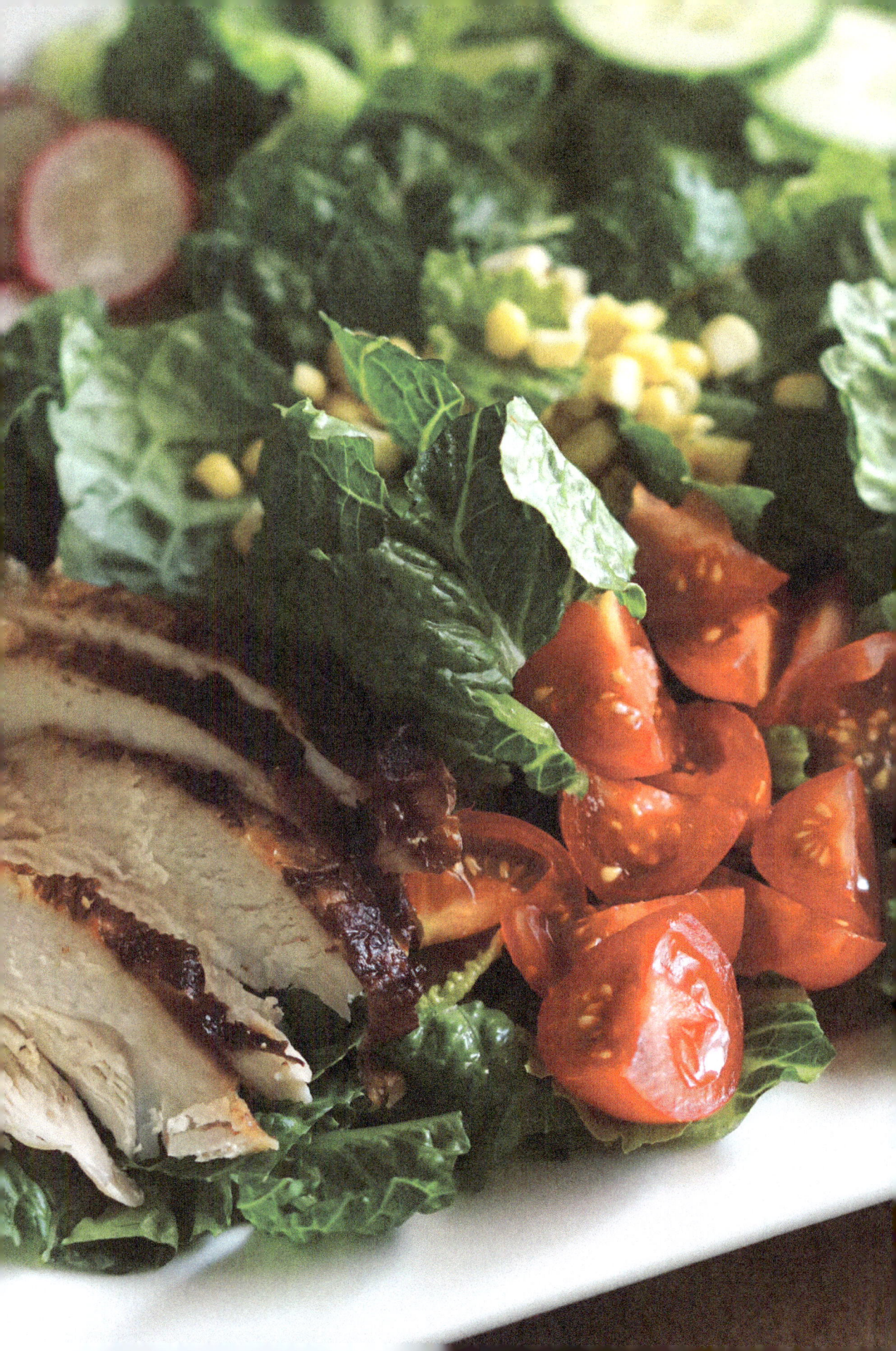

lunch and mains

49 **Kale Salad**
A healthy, delicious way to enjoy one of our favorite superfoods.

50 **Strawberry Avocado Salad**
A refreshing salad, full of healthy fats.

51 **Blackberry Apple Walnut Salad**
A light and colorful salad that is a perfect combination of tangy and sweet.

53 **Cucumber Tomato Salad**
A simple salad, just like grandma used to make.

56 **Shaved Brussels Sprouts Salad**
A raw salad preparation that is great for detoxing.

58 **Detox Salad**
A fresh, organic detox salad that is bursting with nutrition and flavor!

60 **Avocado Soup**
Chilled or hot, this quick soup is a tasty treat.

62 **Kale and Lentil Soup**
One of my favorite fall soups. Perfect with a side of gluten free cornbread.

63 **Turkey Chili**
Healthy, hearty and delicious. What better solution for a cold winter's night?

65 **Red Lentil Soup**
Red lentils cook faster than green or brown lentils so this is a great go-to recipe for lunch on the run or a quick after-work dinner.

67 **Veggie Stir Fry**
Healthy stir fry is a great way to get your veggies in!

69 **Zoodles**
Zucchini noodles (zoodles) are great with avocado dressing or pesto or as a base for spaghetti.

71 **Chicken Salad**
Walnuts, apples, celery, red onion and roasted chicken give this just the right amount of texture and flavor.

73 **Lettuce Wraps**
Butter lettuce piled with your favorite meat and vegetables.

74 **Black Bean Burger**
Try this vegetarian burger on Meatless Monday...or any day of the week.

76 **Burrito Bowl**
Have your favorite Mexican burrito bowl in the comfort of your own home.

78 **Shrimp n Grits**
A favorite Southern dish turned healthy.

79 **Noodle Bowl**
A quick fix meal, ready in 30 minutes or less.

81 **Curried Chicken**
The aroma in your kitchen while making this dish! A very easy chicken recipe, packed with flavor.

83 **Roasted Orange Chicken**
Roasted chicken is great for Sunday dinner or the holidays.

85 **Pan Seared Salmon**
Have you ever had salmon in your favorite restaurant with the crispy skin and wish you could recreate that at home? Here's how!

kale salad

[Serves 2-3]

This kale salad has turned many rabbit food haters into pure kale lovers! I served this as an appetizer to one of my favorite couples, during dinner, and they stared at each other like, "What IS this?" Before they took two bites they were asking me for the recipe and making a grocery list so they could replicate it at home. Coupled with my basic salad dressing, which is my go-to dressing for salads, it is light, it is fast and it is good for you.

1 bunch curly kale, ribs removed
Kosher salt and freshly ground black pepper
1/4 cup almond slivers
1 large red apple, chopped
1/2 cup cucumber slices
1/4 cup red onion, chopped
1 small garlic clove, minced
2 tablespoons turkey bacon bits
1/4 cup unsweetened cranberries, *optional*
Goat cheese crumbles, *optional*

Chop kale into small pieces. Massage kale leaves in Every Day Salad dressing [page 136] until withered. Do not skip this step or the leaves will be tough. Let stand for 10 minutes.

Add salt and pepper, to taste. Combine remaining ingredients and toss until coated. Serve.

strawberry avocado salad

[Serves 2]

When strawberries are in season, this is a great refreshing salad that is filling enough for lunch or dinner. Pair it with my creamy and delicious avocado lime dressing.

6 cups fresh baby spinach
8-10 large strawberries, hulled and sliced
1 small avocado, cut into chunks
1/4 cup goat cheese crumbles
1/4 cup walnuts, toasted
1/2 small red onion, thinly sliced

Gently mix together ingredients in a large salad bowl. Drizzle Avocado Lime dressing [page 138] over salad and toss until salad is evenly coated. Top with goat cheese crumbles. Serve immediately.

Optional: Top with cooked boneless, skinless chicken breast.

blackberry apple walnut salad

[Serves 2]

This blackberry apple walnut salad is refreshing, nutritious and delicious. Pair it with my poppy seed dressing for a light and tangy salad.

6 cups Artisan lettuce, chopped
2 red apples, thinly sliced
1 cup almond slivers
1/2 small red onion, thinly sliced
Half of an English cucumber
1/4 cup goat cheese crumbles
Handful of blackberries
Roasted chicken (optional)

Poppy seed Dressing:
1/2 cup olive oil
3 tablespoons apple cider vinegar
1 teaspoon stevia (or 2 teaspoons raw honey)
1 tablespoon poppy seeds
1 teaspoon ground dry mustard
1/2 teaspoon ginger powder
1/2 teaspoon salt
1/4 teaspoon fresh ground black pepper

Add the lettuce, apples, almonds, onion, cucumber and chicken (optional) together in a large salad bowl.

Drizzle Poppy seed dressing [page 137] over salad and toss until salad is evenly coated. Top with goat cheese crumbles and blackberries. Serve.

Add all ingredients to a mason jar, blender or food processor. Process until smooth. Serve over salad.

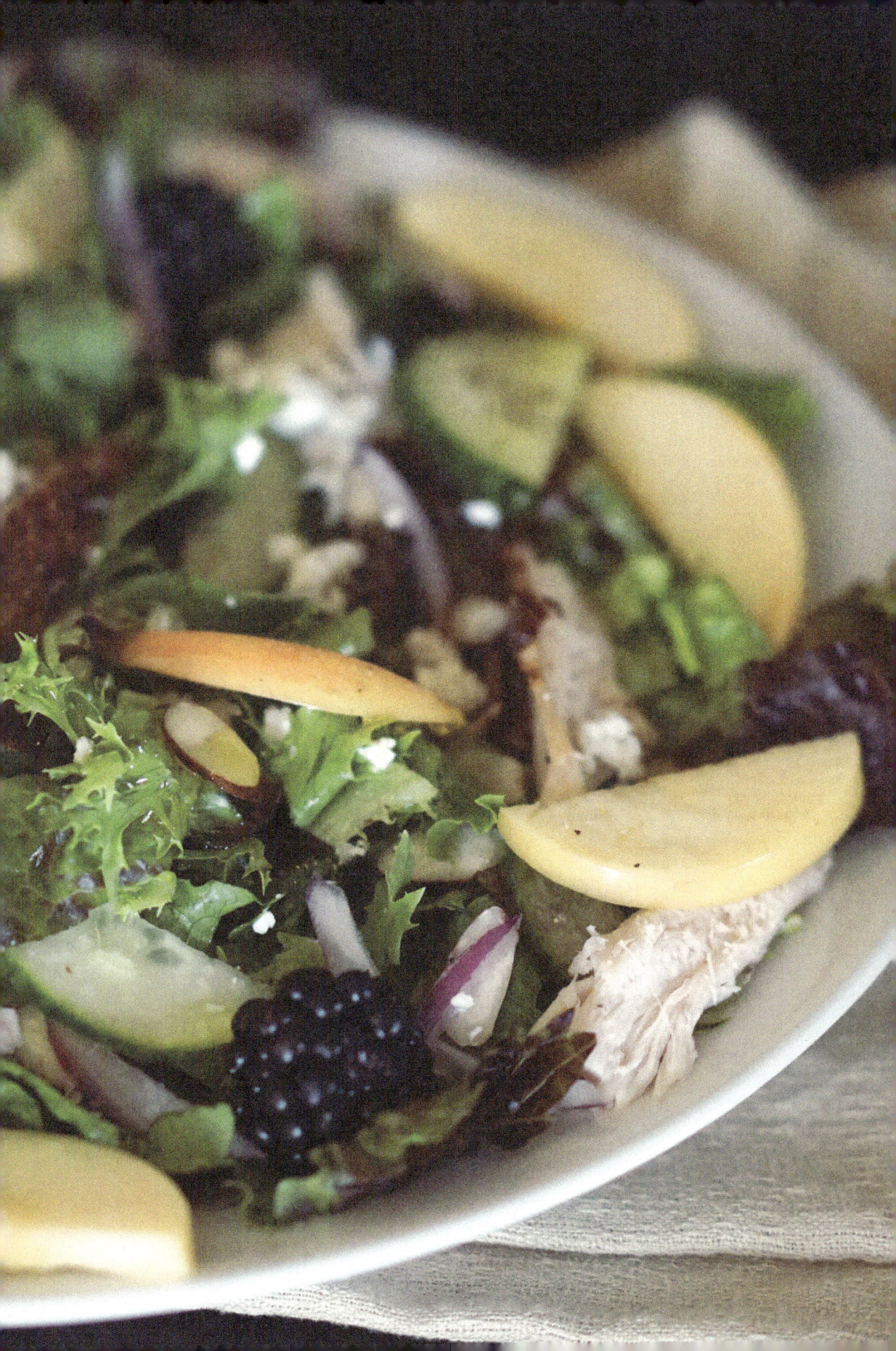

cucumber tomato salad

[Serves 2]

This was a simple dish my grandmother used to make. She would put this in her Tupperware container, grab a fork, and we would sit at the kitchen table eating it until the vinegar was too much to bear. Instead of using white vinegar as she did, substitute organic apple cider vinegar. Takes me back to the good ol' days…

1 carton organic grape tomatoes, halved
Half of small red onion, thinly sliced
1 organic cucumber, thinly sliced
1/4 cup extra-virgin olive oil
2 tablespoons organic apple cider vinegar
1 teaspoon dill
Kosher salt and ground black pepper, to taste

Cut tomatoes in halves lengthwise. Slice the onion and cucumber into thin slices. Mix the olive oil, apple cider vinegar and seasonings in a small bowl until well combined. Add the salad ingredients, toss and serve cold.

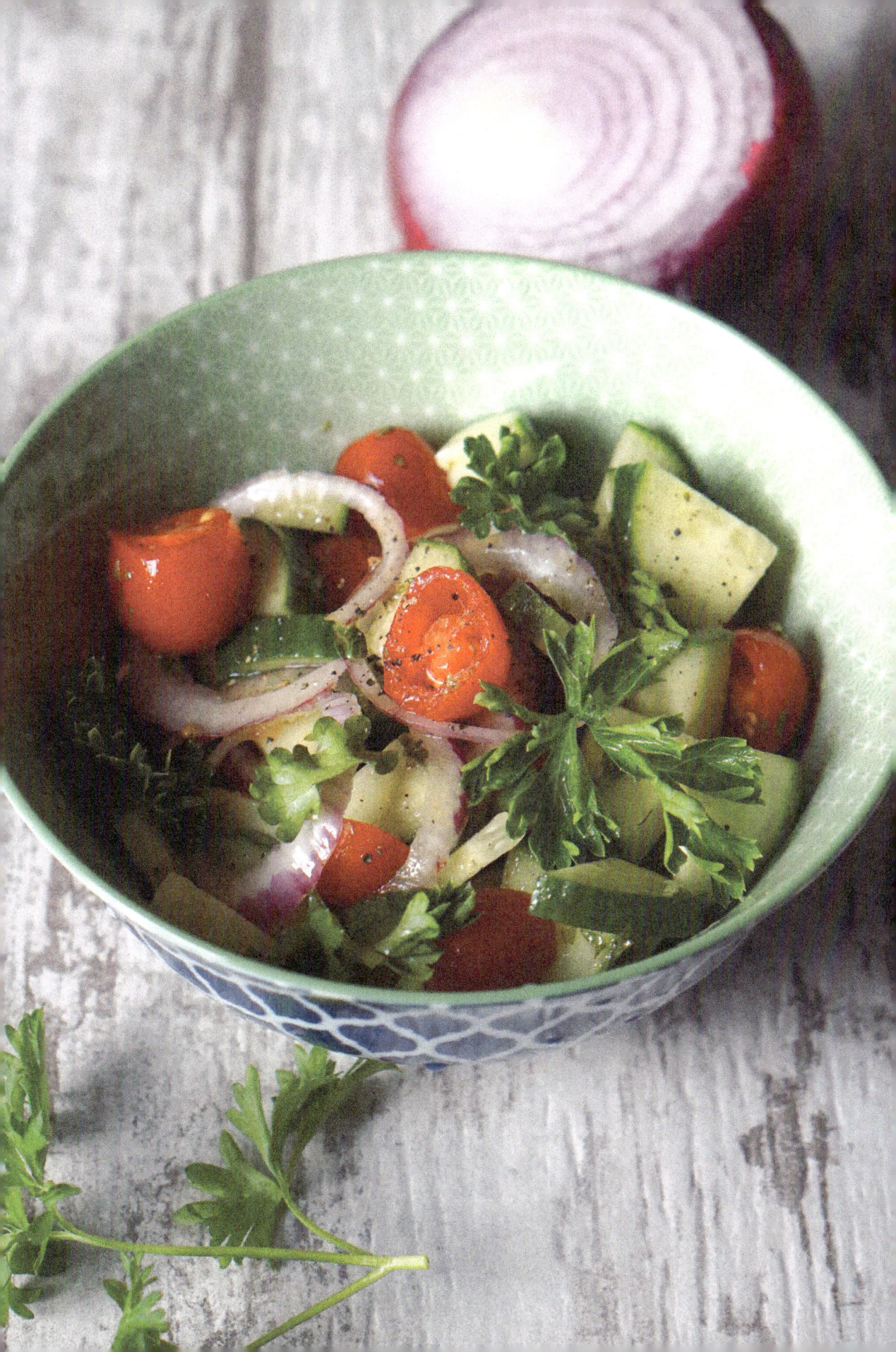

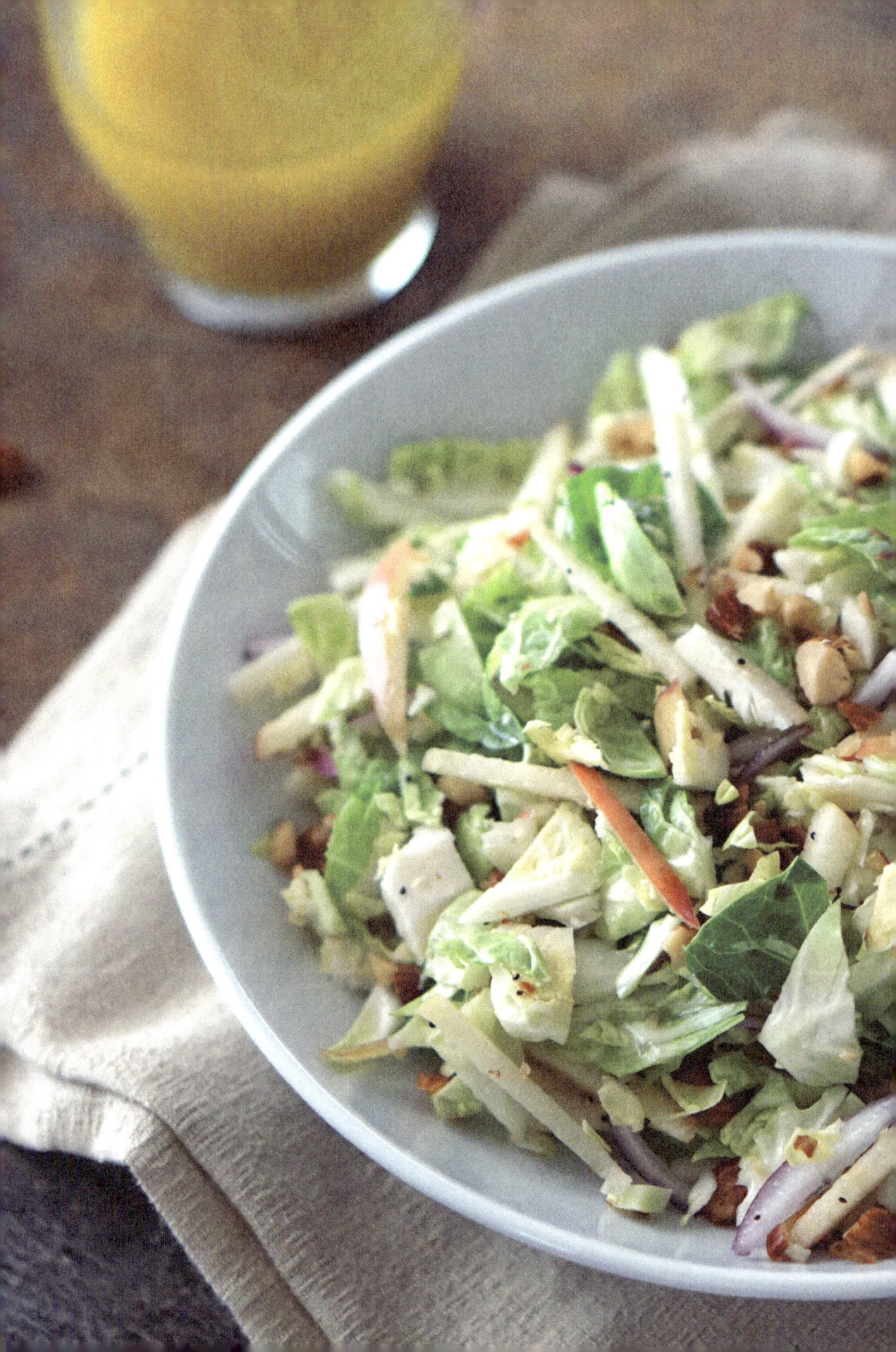

shaved brussels sprouts salad

[Serves 4]

Brussels sprouts are one of my favorite foods and they have a host of valuable benefits that can boost your overall health. If you have never tried Brussels sprouts before, don't let them intimidate you - just think of it like eating cabbage with a twist. Eating them raw is especially great for you as the glucosinates in them are cancer fighters.

1 pound Brussels sprouts
2 red apples
1 medium red onion
2 slices turkey bacon, optional
1 cup chopped almonds

Vinaigrette:
4 tablespoons fresh lemon juice
1/2 cup extra virgin olive oil
2 teaspoons mustard powder
1 dropper liquid stevia
1 clove garlic
Salt and pepper, to taste

Cook the turkey bacon until crisped in a 425 degree oven. Cool and set aside.

Trim the ends off of the Brussels sprouts. Using a sharp knife or a mandolin, shave the sprouts. Chop the apples, red onion, and turkey bacon. Combine in a large bowl.

Toast the almonds in a skillet over medium-high heat, stirring frequently, until fragrant, about two minutes. Add to the Brussels sprout mixture. Toss to combine.

Combine the vinaigrette ingredients in a mini food processor. Pour some of the dressing over the salad mixture and toss to coat.

.....
This salad is also great with fresh, organic peaches
(instead of apples).

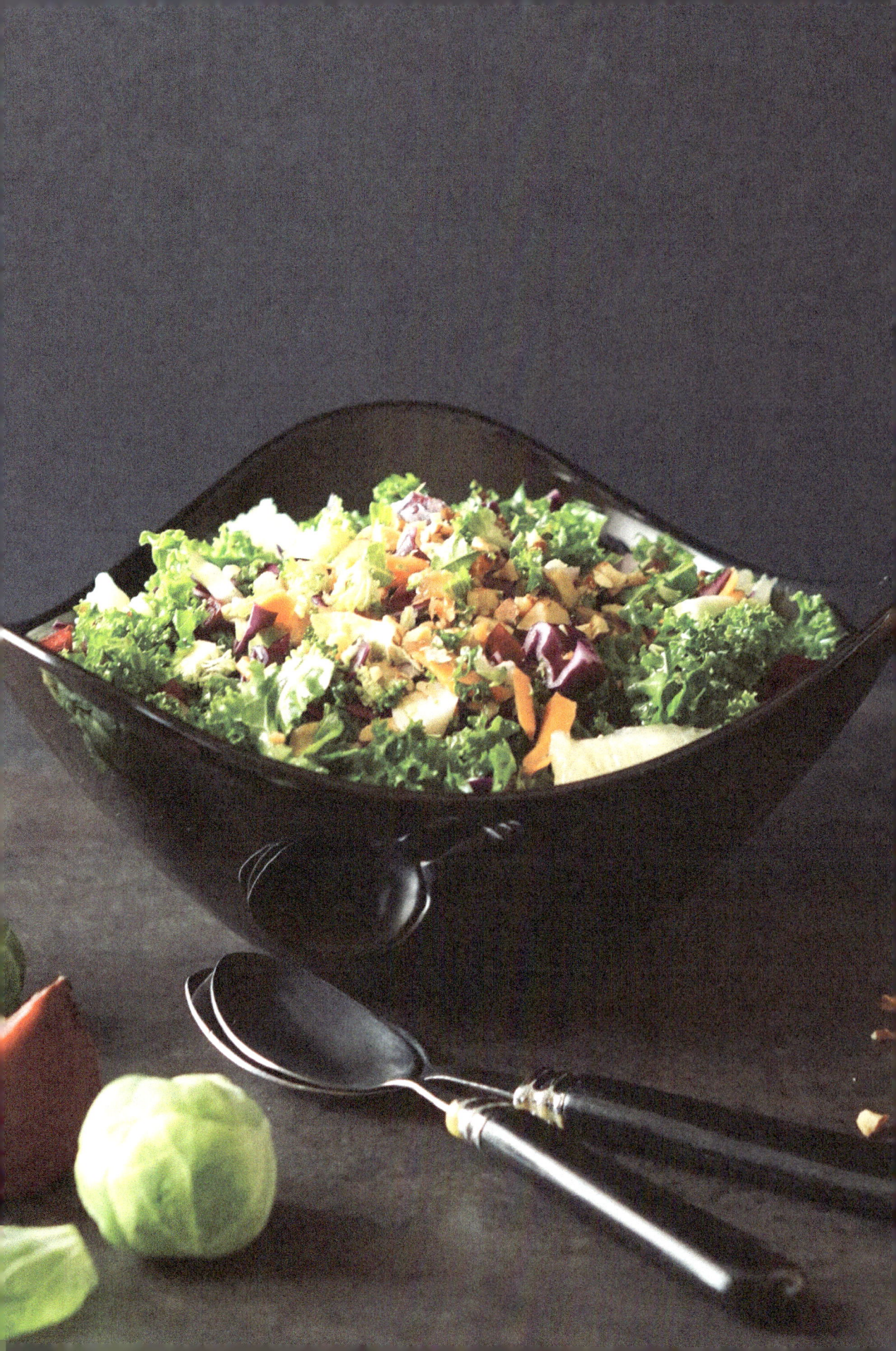

detox salad

[Serves 2-3]

Because I have Lyme Disease, I have a lot of issues with toxin overload. When my system is overburdened, I typically get signs like excessive congestion, frequent headaches, bloating and rashes on my skin. In these times I do more juicing and eating raw preparations like this detox salad. A great and gentle way to cleanse the liver naturally.

Salad:
1/2 cup toasted almonds
2 cups kale
2 cups broccoli florets
2 cups Brussels sprouts
2 cups red cabbage
1 cup carrots
1 small red onion
1 cup organic beets
1 pink grapefruit, peeled and segmented

Dressing:
4 tablespoons fresh lemon juice
1/2 cup extra virgin olive oil
1 dropper liquid stevia
1 clove garlic
Salt and pepper, to taste

Toasted Almonds:
Preheat the oven to 350 degrees. Place nuts in a single layer on a rimmed baking sheet. Bake 5-7 minutes until they are golden brown. Set aside to cool.

For the Salad:
Using a food processor, process the kale, broccoli, Brussels sprouts, cabbage, carrots and onions until chopped. Add to a large bowl.

Rough chop the almonds, dice the beets and add them, along with the grapefruit pieces, to the chopped salad ingredients.

Add the dressing ingredients to a mini food processor. Blend until processed. Pour over salad and toss.

avocado soup

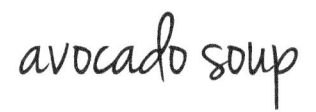

[Serves 2]

This creamy, luscious soup is a quick appetizer or lunch item. Can be served chilled or slightly warm. A quick and easy dish made in the blender.

1/2 large English cucumber
2 large avocados
1 garlic clove, minced
1/2 cup water
1 1/2 organic chicken stock
Salt and pepper to taste
Dash of fresh lime juice

For the corn salsa:
1 ear of sweet corn
1/4 cup red onion
1/2 teaspoon extra virgin olive oil

Preheat oven to 425 degrees.

Rub a little olive oil on corn and wrap in foil. Roast the ear of corn on a cookie sheet for about 20 minutes. Allow corn to cool. Remove the kernels and place in a large bowl. Add onion and parsley and toss with olive oil. Set aside.

Peel the cucumber and cut in into smaller pieces. Peel and pit the avocado. Cut flesh into chunks. In a food processor or blender, add the cucumber, avocado, garlic, water, chicken stock and seasonings. Pulse until the mixture is smooth or select the soup option on your blender, if the option is available.

Taste the soup and adjust seasoning, if necessary. Serve chilled.

Optional: Garnish with corn salsa.

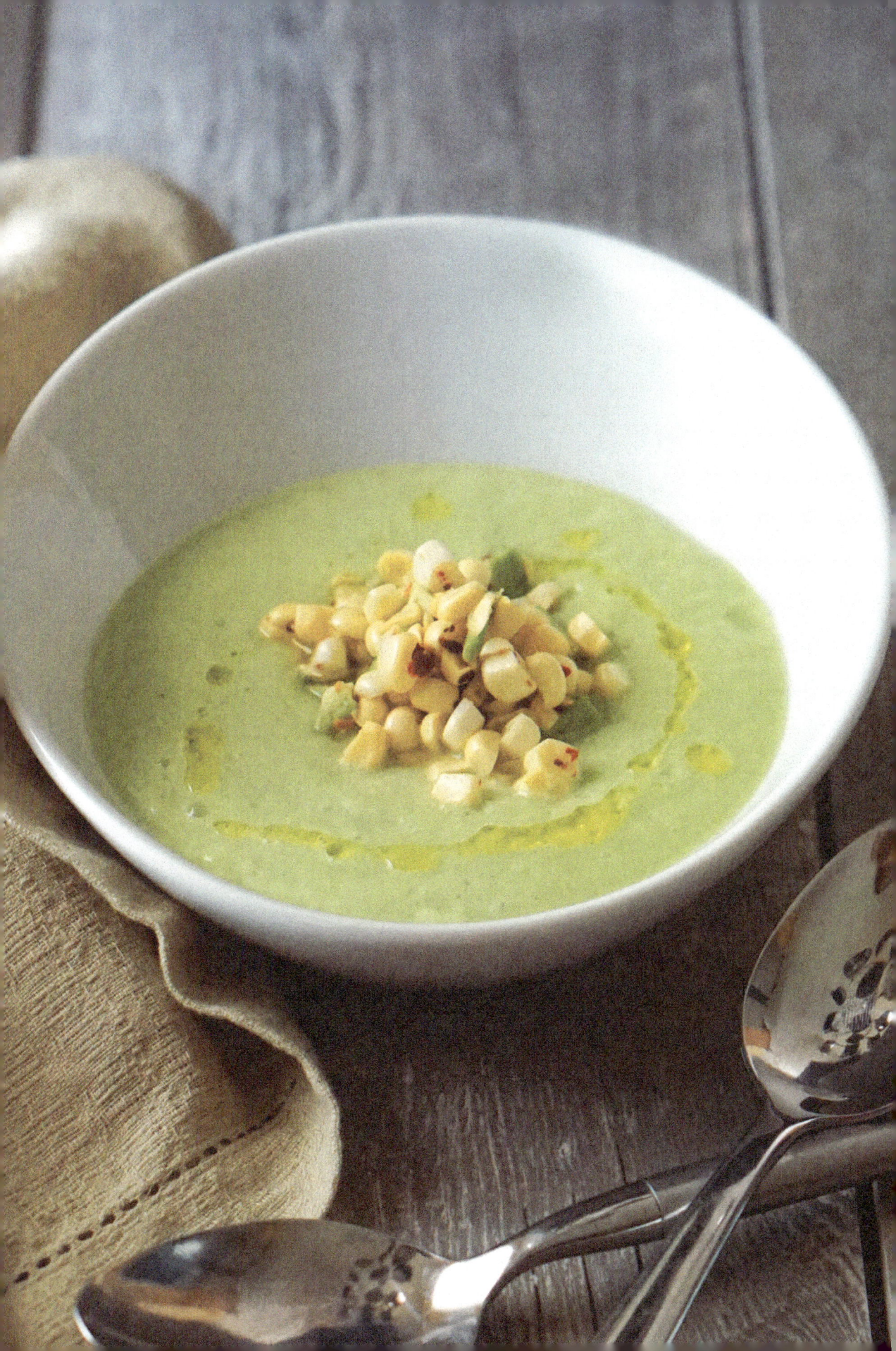

kale and lentil soup

[Serves 2-3]

I love a good, hearty soup and will eat soup year round. But this soup reminds me of fall with the sweet potatoes and the chicken apple sausage. Simply delicious!

1 tablespoon olive oil
1 medium onion, diced
2 stalks of celery, diced
1 clove fresh garlic
1 cup dry brown or green lentils, rinsed
4 cups chicken stock
1/2 cup water
1 organic tomato, pureed
1 teaspoon kosher salt
1 teaspoon ground black pepper
1/4 teaspoon cumin
1/4 teaspoon paprika
Fresh parsley
1 medium sweet potato, diced
Handful of curly kale, chopped
Cooked chicken apple sausage, optional

Heat olive oil in a heavy-bottomed pot over medium heat. Add onion and celery and saute until softened. Add garlic and saute for an additional minute.

Add lentils, stock, water, tomato puree, herbs and seasonings. Stir together and bring to a boil. Once soup has reached a boil, reduce heat to low and simmer, covered for 20-30 minutes or until lentils are tender.

Add sweet potatoes (and chicken sausage, if using) and simmer until potatoes are tender. In the final minutes of cooking, add kale and simmer, uncovered, just until kale is wilted.

Remove from heat and adjust seasonings, if needed.

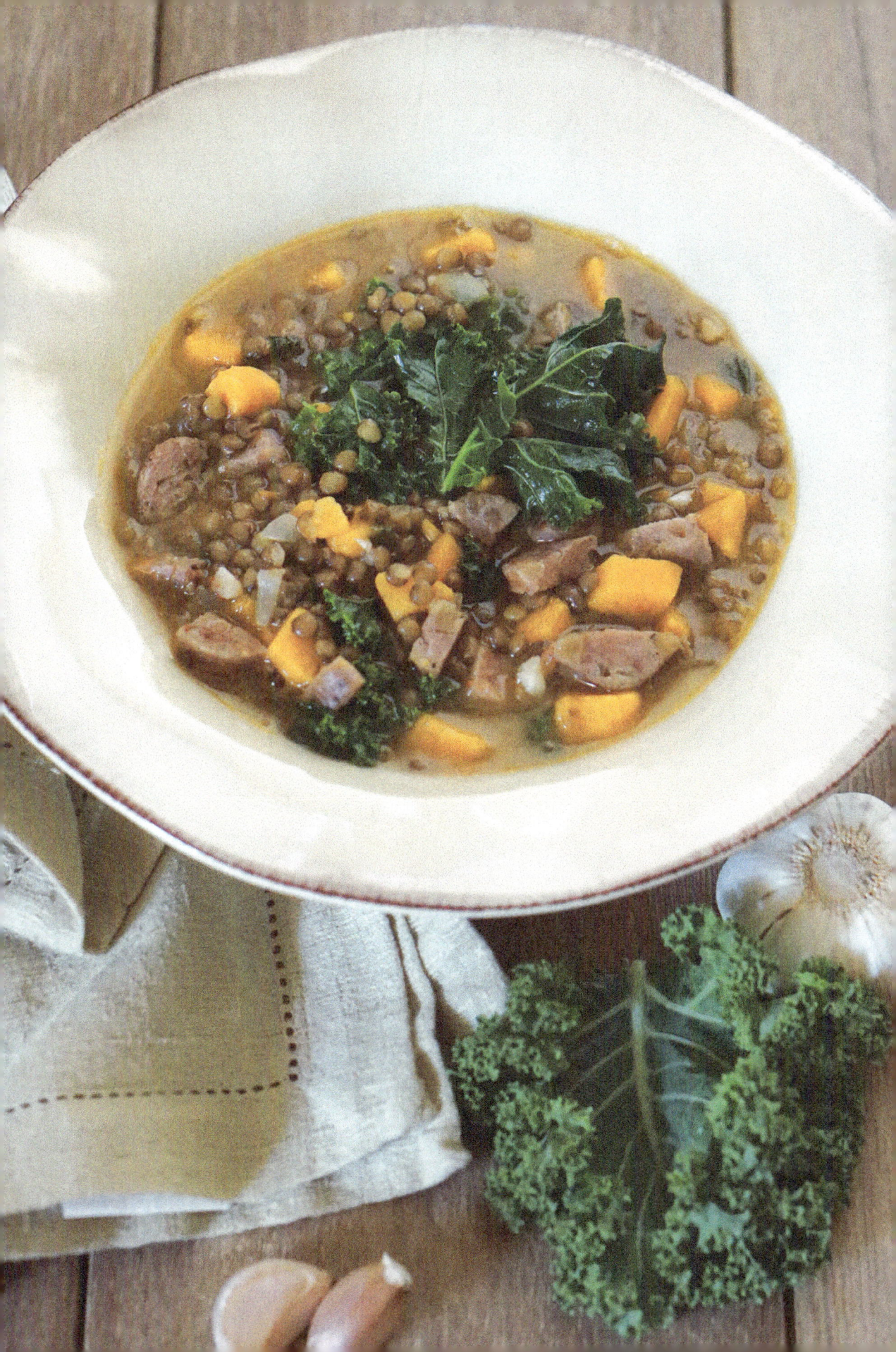

turkey chili

[Serves 4 to 6]

Chili is one of the only things I like about the cold weather. I probably eat chili at least once every other week during the winter months. And there are some foods that just go together - like meatloaf and mashed potatoes, barbeque and slaw, turkey and dressing, ham and macaroni and cheese...ok, ok you get my drift. Well, there is nothing like a bowl of chili with some gluten free skillet cornbread. A marriage made in heaven.

2 tablespoons olive oil
1 pound ground turkey
1 medium yellow onion, diced
1 green pepper, diced
1 red pepper, diced
3/4 cup diced celery
1 large jalapeno pepper, seeded and minced
2 cloves garlic, minced
1/4 cup arrowroot starch/flour
3 tablespoons hot Mexican-style chili powder
1 teaspoon ground cumin
2 teaspoons smoked paprika
1 1/2 teaspoons salt
1/2 to 1 teaspoon cayenne pepper
1 tablespoon organic apple cider vinegar
14-oz organic diced tomatoes with juice
4 cups chicken stock
15-oz organic pinto beans
15-oz organic black beans
15-oz organic garbanzo beans

In a large stock pot, add olive oil and crumble in turkey; add in the onion, peppers, celery, jalapeno and garlic and cook until softened and until turkey is no longer pink. Add the arrowroot flour and combine.

Stir in the seasonings, along with the apple cider vinegar, tomatoes, and chicken stock. Add beans to the pot, with their juices. Bring to a boil. Reduce heat to low, cover and simmer for 45 minutes.

Remove from heat and serve.

Garnish with herbs, scallions, jalapenos, cheese or coconut sour cream.

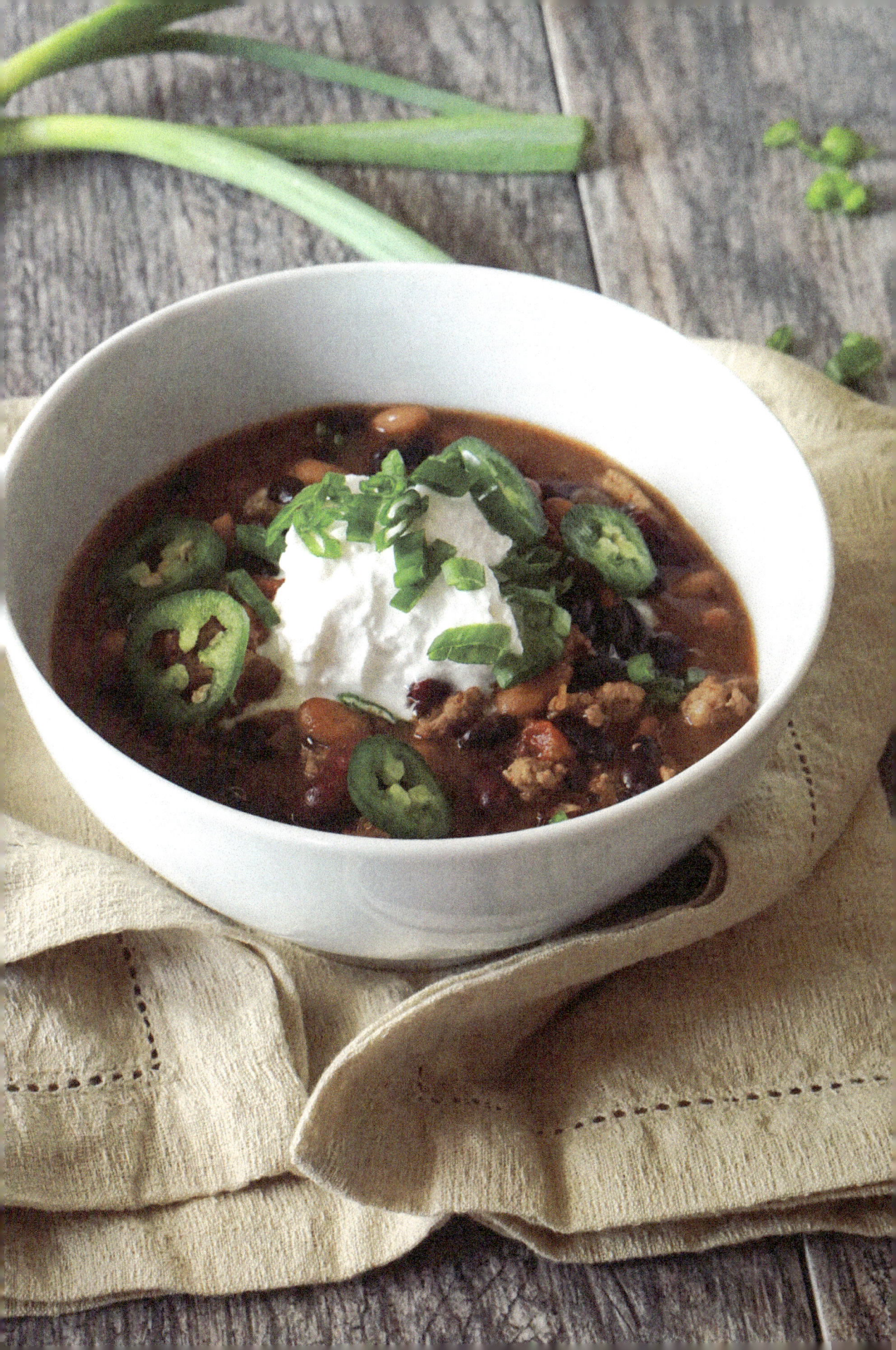

red lentil soup

[Serves 2]

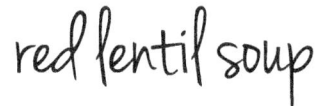

I particularly love red lentils. They cook much faster than their counterparts and are perfect in pureed soups. Red lentils are high in protein so this is a very filling, delicious dish.

1 tablespoon olive oil
1 small yellow onion, diced
2 cloves garlic, minced
2 stalks of celery, chopped
3 cups water
1 cup organic chicken stock
1 cup red lentils
1 teaspoon red pepper flakes
1 teaspoon cumin
1 1/2 teaspoons salt
1/2 teaspoon freshly ground black pepper
1/2 teaspoon turmeric

Fresh cilantro for garnish

In a large pot, heat olive oil over medium high heat. Add onion, garlic, and celery and saute until golden, about 3-5 minutes.

Add seasonings and saute for an additional minute or two.

Add liquids and lentils. Bring to a simmer, then partially cover pot and turn heat to medium-low. Simmer until lentils are soft, about 30 minutes.

Using an immersion blender or a food processor, purée half the soup then add it back to pot. Stir well.

Serve with fresh cilantro or a drizzle of coconut cream.

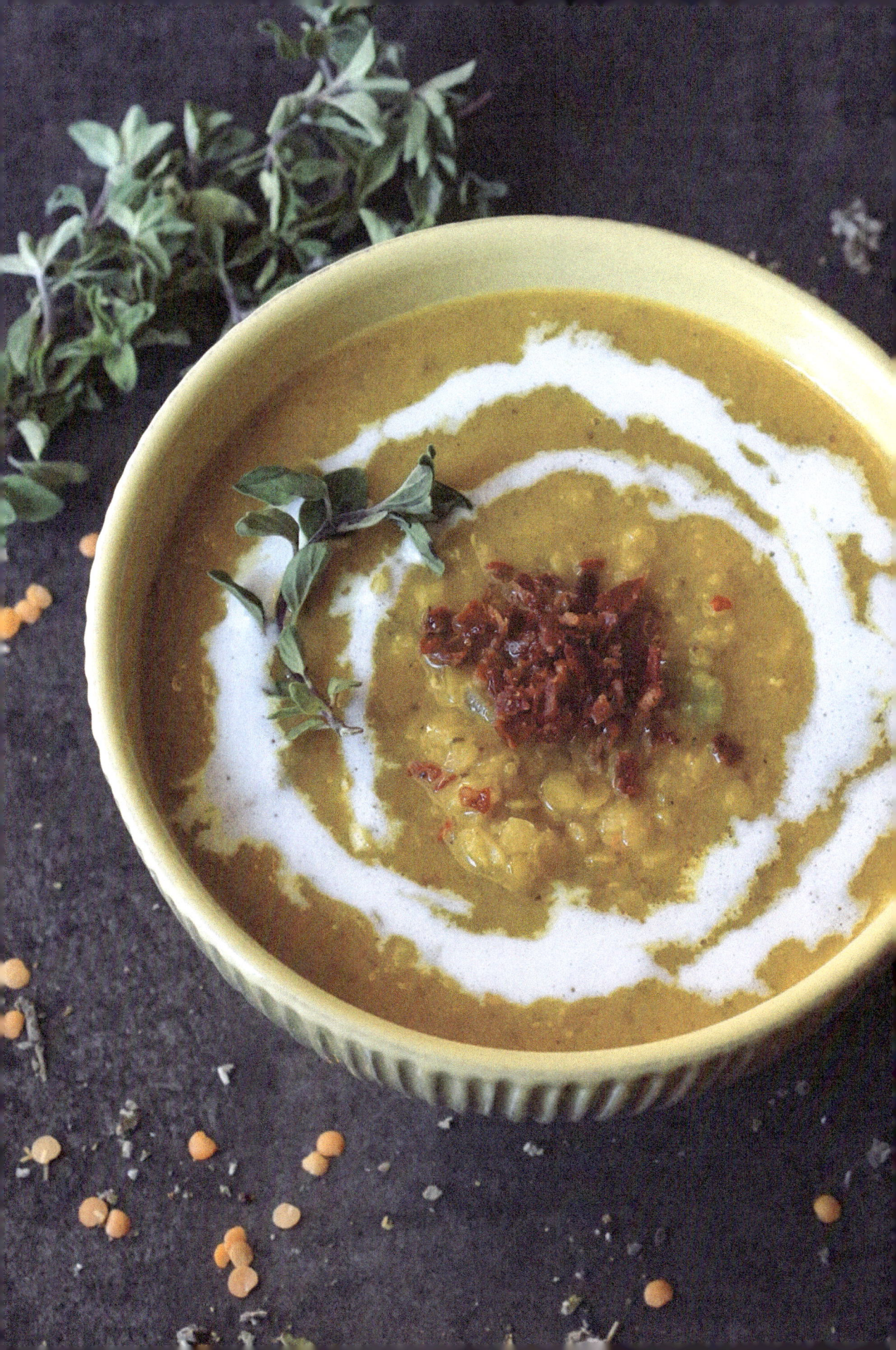

veggie stir fry

[Serves 2]

This colorful dish is packed with all of your favorite vegetables. You don't need a wok to have stir fry at home. If you have a large pan or skillet you can create this dish in minutes. Great for a quick lunch or dinner when you are on the run.

2 tablespoons olive oil, divided
2 cloves garlic, minced
2 large carrots, peeled and julienned
1 large red bell pepper, julienned
1 large green bell pepper, julienned
1 cup snow peas
1 cup shiitake mushrooms, sliced thinly
2 cups fresh broccoli florets
1 small red onion
1/2 yellow squash, *optional*
2 cups cooked brown rice
1/4 to 1/2 cup coconut aminos
Scallions, for garnish

Prepare all vegetables.

Heat a wok or a large saute pan over medium heat with the olive oil. Add the garlic and cook for 2 minutes. Remove from pan and set aside.

Add remaining oil to pan and place over medium-high heat. Once hot, add the vegetables and cook, stirring frequently, for about 6-8 minutes. [You still want vegetables to be crunchy and vibrant in color].

Add brown rice to pan and stir frequently. Pour coconut aminos over mixture and toss. Serve hot.

Optional: Add cooked chicken or shrimp.

Alternate Sauce for Stir Fry:

3 tablespoons tahini or almond butter
3 tablespoons coconut aminos
3 tablespoons freshly squeezed orange juice
1 drop liquid stevia
1 teaspoon grated fresh ginger

Use one or two day old rice for stir-fry. If you use rice made the same day, your dish will turn out mushy.

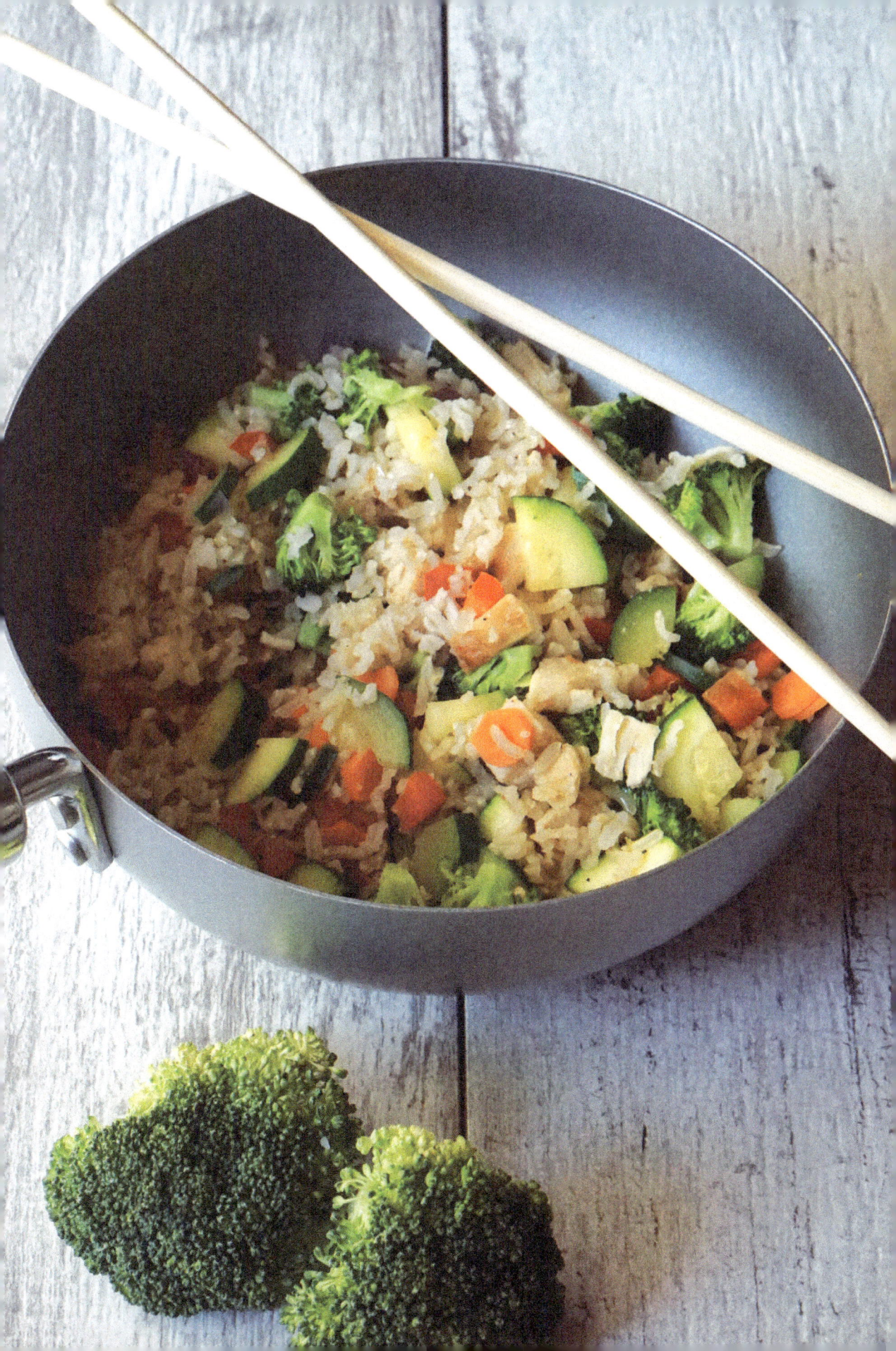

zoodles

[Serves 2]

I started eating zoodles when I was practicing eating a raw diet and fell in love with them. Zoodles can be eaten as a salad or a main dish and are good hot or cold. Try substituting your spaghetti noodles with zoodles for a healthier alternative...or toss them in some pesto, my fave!

1 large zucchini squash
2 cups fresh basil or kale
2-3 tablespoons olive oil
1-2 cloves fresh garlic
1/4 teaspoon sea salt
1/4 cup pine nuts or walnuts

Use a spiralizer or julienne peeler to spiralize your zucchini squash into noodles.

Place basil (or kale) in a mini food processor and pulse to finely chop leaves. Add remaining ingredients in a food processor and process until smooth.

Toss pesto with zucchini noodles (zoodles) and serve. *Optional: Garnish zoodles with additional pine nuts and grape tomatoes.*

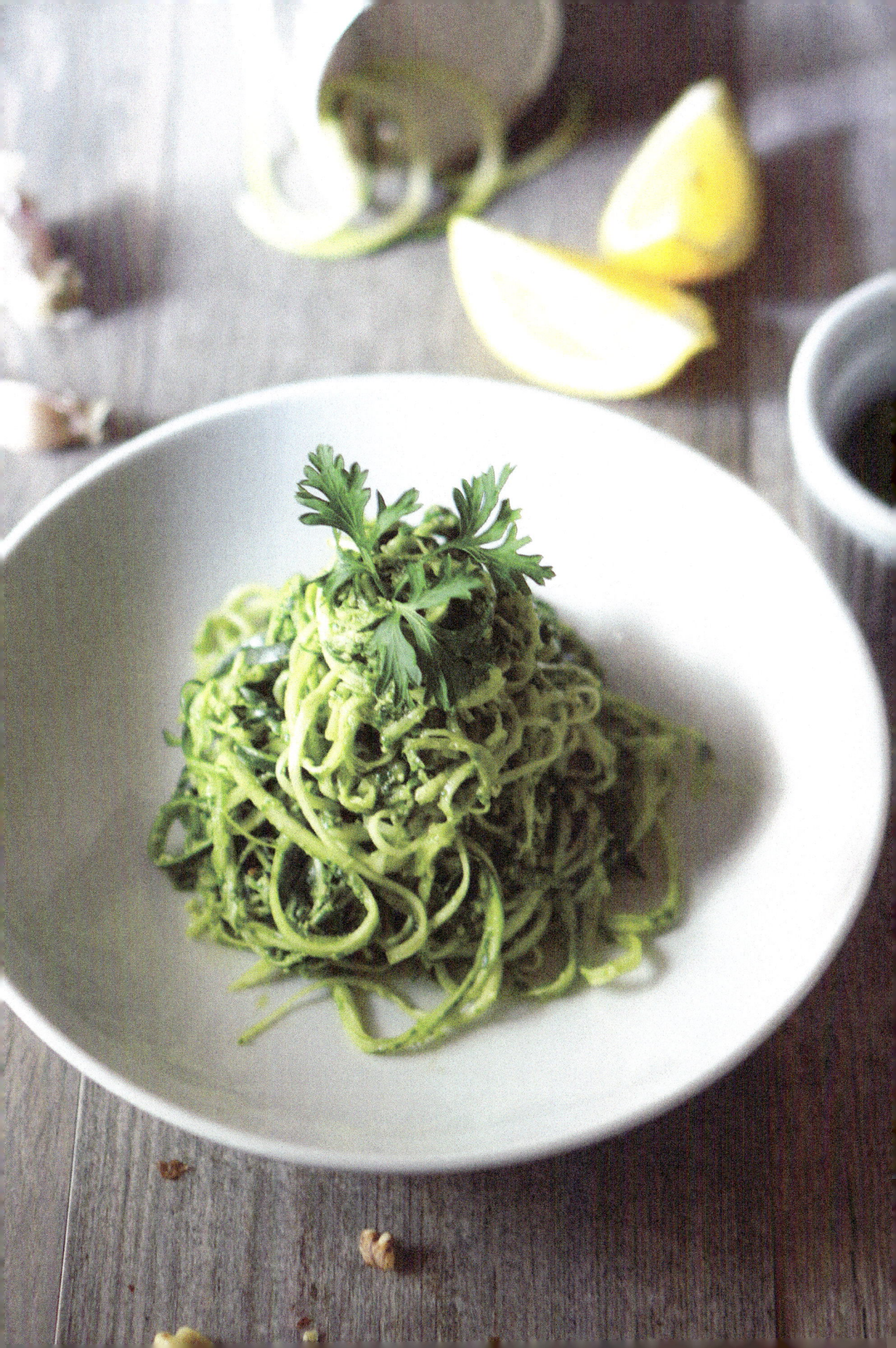

chicken salad

[Serves 2]

In a rush? You can make this chicken salad with shredded leftover chicken, store bought chicken roasters, or boneless skinless chicken breasts. If you do not have time to make your own mayonnaise, take some coconut cream, whip it and add a tiny bit of stevia. Substitute that as the mayonnaise in this dish. You will hardly miss it!

3 cups cooked organic chicken, chopped
2 stalks chopped celery
1/4 cup red onion, chopped
1 cup red apple, diced
1/3 cup toasted walnuts, chopped
3/4 cup mayonnaise
2 teaspoons poppy seeds
1 teaspoon of organic apple cider vinegar or fresh lemon juice
Dash of liquid stevia, optional
Salt and pepper to taste

For the mayonnaise:

[See recipe on page 140]

For the chicken salad:

In a large mixing bowl, add the chicken, celery, onion, apples and toasted walnuts. Add the mayonnaise and toss until combined. Add the poppy seeds, apple cider vinegar, stevia and salt and pepper. Adjust seasoning to your liking and serve.

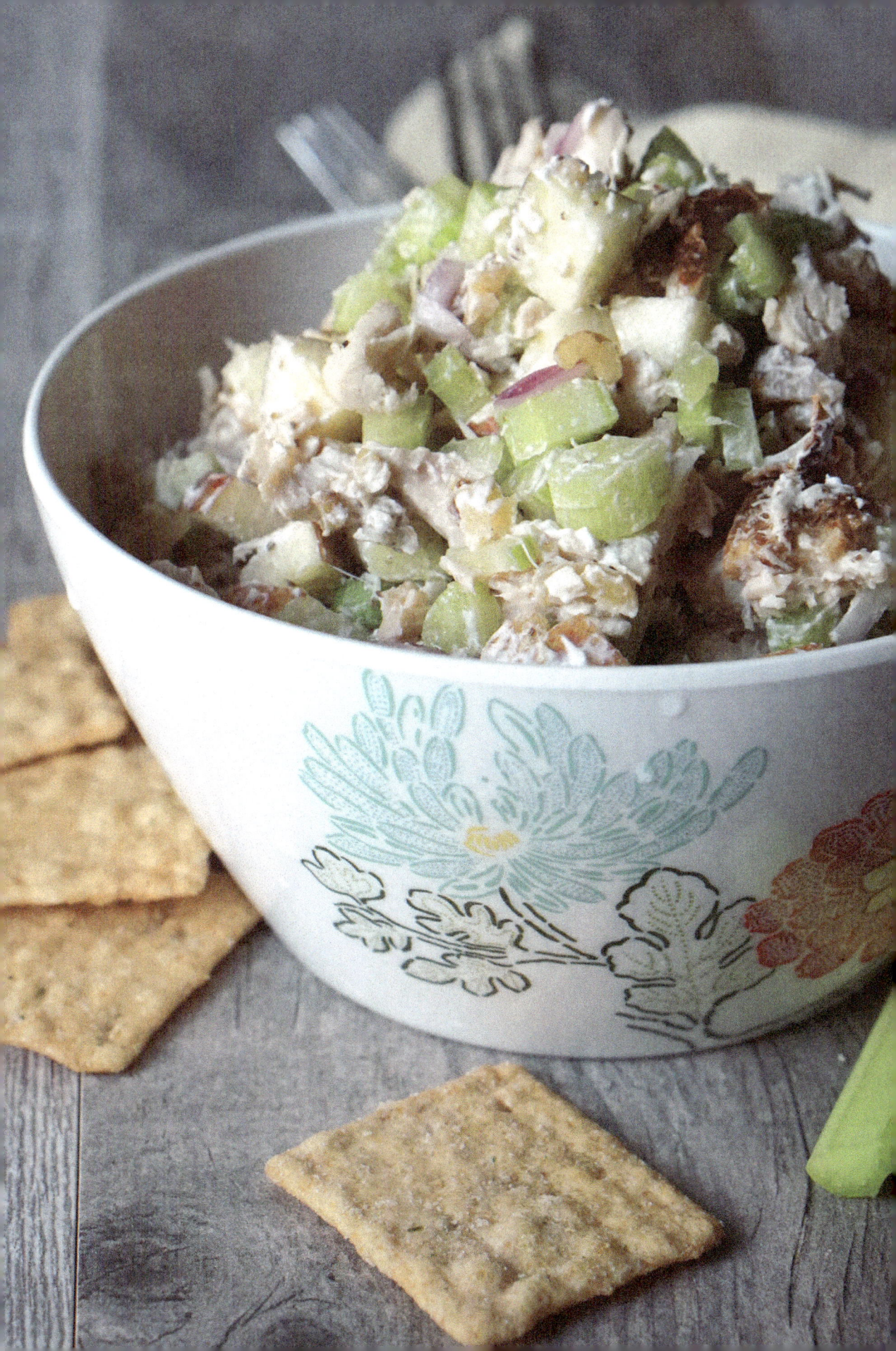

lettuce wraps

[Serves 2]

Just like with a taco, I can eat ten of these wraps and they are never enough. Yes, ten! Hey, you can do that when you eat a lot of foods with no calories. Use ground turkey, ground beef or diced chicken breasts as your protein. The rest really just depends on what is in the fridge. Have fun with it!

1 tablespoon olive oil
1 pound ground turkey
2 cloves garlic, minced
1 onion, diced
1/4 cup coconut aminos
Salt and pepper, to taste
1/2 cup cucumber, diced
1/4 cup fresh peaches, cut into chunks
1/4 cup red tomatoes, diced
2 scallions, thinly sliced
1 head butter lettuce

Heat olive oil in a saucepan over medium high heat. Add ground turkey meat, crumbled, and cook until browned, about 3-5 minutes.

Stir in garlic, onion, and coconut aminos and cook until onions have become translucent, about 2-3 minutes. Season with salt and pepper, to taste. Mix well.

In a medium sized bowl, combine cucumber, peaches, tomatoes and scallions.

To serve, spoon several tablespoons of the meat and the toppings into the lettuce leaf, taco style.

black bean burger

[Serves 2]

Meatless Mondays no longer have to be a bore. This is a very satisfying dish with a meaty texture that can be patted out ahead of time and made at your convenience. If you don't have any brown rice on hand, use leftover quinoa. And if you want an even more filling dish, add a bit of mashed sweet potato.

2 cups canned organic black beans, rinsed
1 small yellow onion, chopped
1 garlic clove, minced
2-3 scallions, chopped
1 teaspoon cumin
1 teaspoon chili powder
1 teaspoon smoked paprika
Salt and pepper to taste
1 1/4 cup leftover cooked brown rice

Drain the beans, rinse them and mash them with a spoon in a large bowl. Set aside.

In a skillet saute the onions, garlic, scallions and spices until translucent. Add this mixture, along with the cooked rice, to the beans. Using your hands, mix well.

Divide the mixture into equal parts, to make about 6 burger patties. Shape them into rounds and put them on a baking tray. Heat a skillet over medium heat and add the patties to the pan. State patties on both sides until cooked through, about 3-5 minutes on each side.

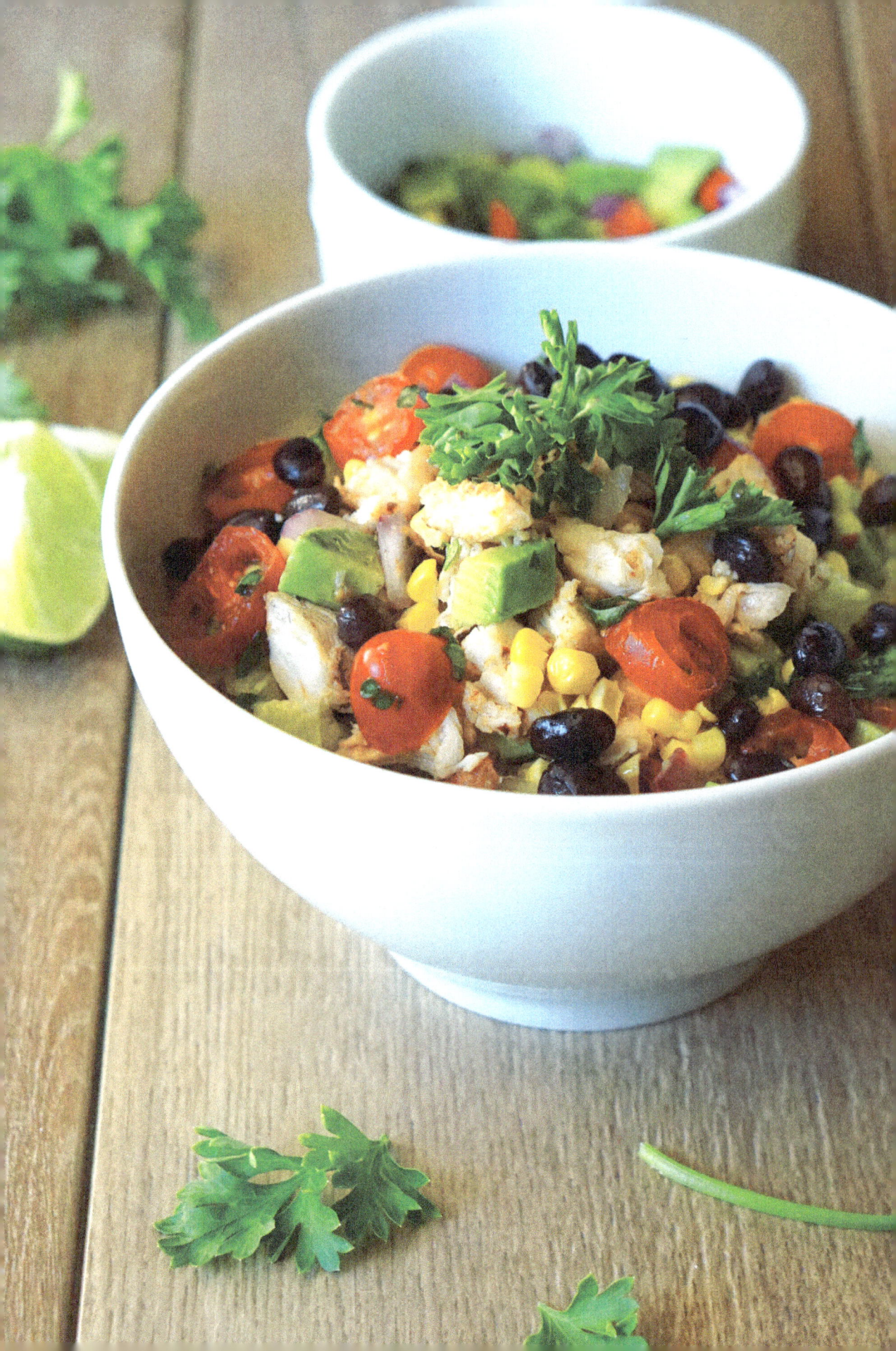

burrito bowl

[Serves 2-3]

Chipot.....whaaaaat???? YOU, yes you, can make your own DIY burrito bowls in the comfort of your own kitchen. With the long list of ingredients it looks like it will take hours to make but it is really very simple.

Rice:
2 cups cooked brown basmati rice
1/4 cup fresh cilantro, chopped
juice of one lime

Chicken:
2 boneless skinless chicken breasts
1 tablespoon olive oil
Kosher salt and ground black pepper
Smoked paprika

Fajita Veggies:
2 teaspoons olive oil
1 large green pepper, sliced
1 red onion, peeled and sliced

Additional burrito bowl Ingredients:
1 cup of cooked black beans
1 cup chopped Romaine lettuce
2 scallions chopped

Corn Salsa:
2 cups of fresh, organic corn
1/4 cup red onion, diced
2 teaspoons chopped cilantro
1/2 cup fresh tomatoes, diced
Dash of fresh lime juice

Cilantro, for garnish

For the rice:
In a large bowl, combine the rice, cilantro and lime juice. Set aside.

For the chicken:
Rub the chicken breasts with olive oil on both sides. Season the chicken breasts with salt, pepper and smoked paprika. Heat a cast iron skillet on medium high heat. Brown chicken breasts on both sides, about 2 minutes per side. Cook chicken, covered, for 15-20 minutes or until chicken is no longer pink and is cooked through. Remove from heat and let the chicken rest. Once cooled, cut into chunks.

For the fajita veggies:
In a saute pan, add 2 teaspoons of olive oil. Add green peppers and onions. Saute for 5-7 minutes, until softened. Set aside.

For the corn salsa:
Toss the ingredients until combined.

To assemble the burrito bowls:
Portion the cilantro brown rice between serving bowls. Divide the remaining ingredients, between the bowls, on top of the rice.

Top with corn salsa.

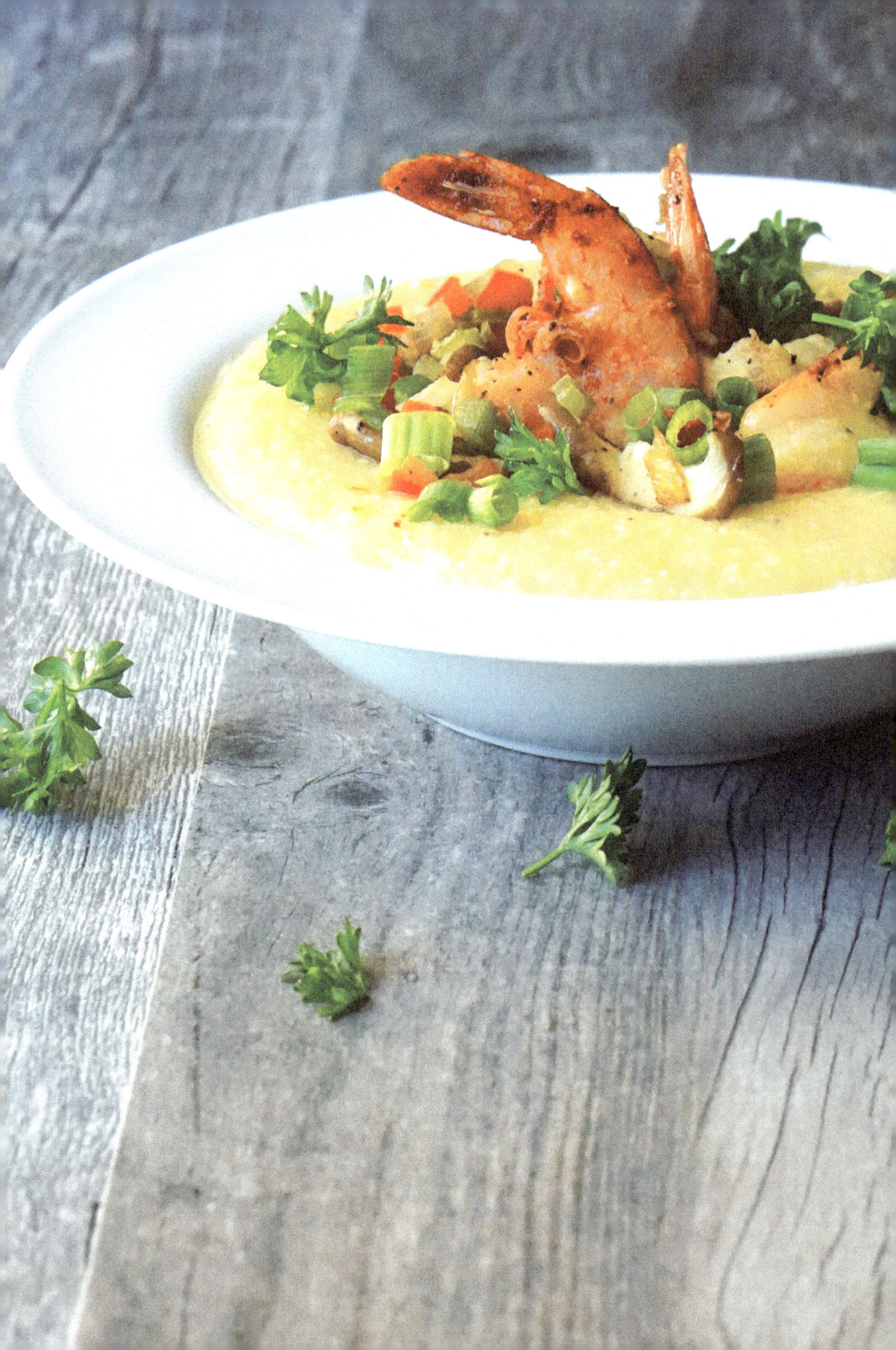

shrimp n' grits

[Serves 2]

When I could eat refined carbs, I loved to eat grits for breakfast. But I enjoy polenta more with savory meals, such as fish and shrimp and grits. Polenta is just cornmeal simmered in water or chicken stock to create a thick, porridge-like, creamy mixture. Pour it into a shallow pan, lined with parchment paper, and allow to cool if you want to eat it in squares. Or you can simply eat it with butter, like a bowl of grits.

2 teaspoons extra virgin olive oil
1/4 cup red onion, chopped
2 cloves garlic, minced
2 cups organic chicken stock
2 cups water
1 1/2 teaspoon kosher salt
1/4 teaspoon ground black pepper
1 cup corn grits, polenta
2 tablespoons butter

1 pound large shrimp, peeled and deveined
Salt and pepper, to taste
Smoked paprika
1-2 tablespoons olive oil
1/2 cup shiitake mushrooms, thinly sliced
1/2 cup green peppers, chopped
1/2 cup red peppers, chopped
1 garlic clove, minced
3/4 cup organic chicken stock
1 tablespoon fresh lemon juice
1 tablespoon butter

Scallions
4 slices cooked turkey bacon (chopped), *optional*

For the polenta:
Heat the olive oil over medium heat. Add the red onion and garlic and cook until onion turns translucent. Add the chicken stock, water, and salt and pepper. Increase the heat, and bring liquids to a boil. Gradually whisk in the corn grits. Cover and cook for 30-40 minutes, stirring every few minutes to prevent lumps. Add butter. Set aside.

For the Shrimp n Grits:

Lightly season shrimp with salt, pepper and smoked paprika. Over medium-high heat, add shrimp to skillet and cook, turning once, until bright pink. Transfer shrimp to a plate. Set aside.

Lower heat, add mushrooms and peppers to skillet and cook for approximately 5 minutes. Add garlic and cook approximately 1 minute more. Increase heat, add chicken stock, and scrape bottom of skillet with a wooden spoon. Cook until stock reduces. Return shrimp to skillet along with the lemon juice and butter, and cook for a minute, until sauce thickens.

Ladle shrimp and sauce over polenta and garnish with scallions, bacon and fresh herbs if desired.

noodle bowl

[Serves 2]

Noodle bowls are very versatile. You can substitute your favorite vegetables and even make it with lamb or beef, if your diet allows.

2 boiled eggs
1 ear of corn, roasted
1-2 tablespoons olive oil
1/2 cup carrots, chopped
1 cup shiitake mushrooms, chopped
1/2 cup broccoli
1 cup snow peas
2 cloves garlic, minced
1 teaspoon salt
1/2 teaspoon pepper
2 cups organic chicken stock
1 cup water
1/2 cup coconut aminos
4 ounces dry noodles
10 shrimp, peeled and deveined
Salt and freshly ground black pepper, to taste
Smoked paprika

Boil two eggs in a pot until done. Set aside.

Preheat oven to 425 degrees. Rub a little olive oil on corn and wrap in foil. Roast the ears of corn on a cookie sheet for about 20 minutes. Allow corn to cool. Remove the kernels and set aside.

In a large heavy bottom pot saute carrots, mushrooms, broccoli and snow peas in olive oil over medium heat for two minutes. Add garlic. State 2-3 minutes, stirring often. Add seasonings and cook for another 2 minutes. Set aside.

In a separate pot, add chicken stock, water and coconut aminos and bring to a boil. Once boiling, add pasta. Bring to a boil once more, turn heat to medium, and simmer until pasta is done.

Season the shrimp with salt, pepper and smoked paprika. While pasta is cooking, broil shrimp on high for 5-7 minutes in the oven or until no longer pink. Set aside.

Assemble bowls by placing noodles, cooked vegetables and protein in a large bowl. Pour stock over the bowl contents.

Garnish with fresh herbs and scallions.

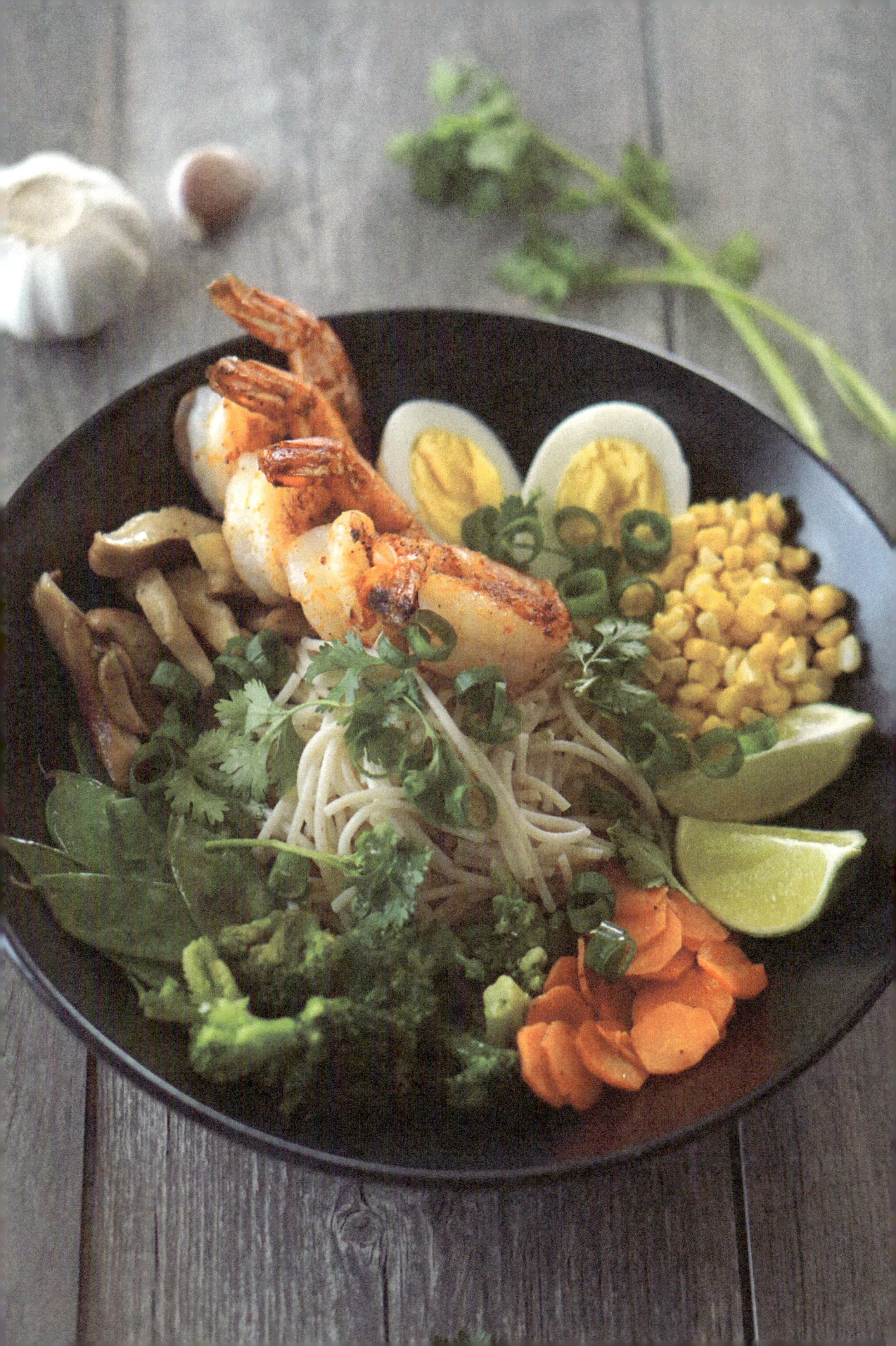

curried chicken

[Serves 2-3]

The smell in the kitchen when this dish is cooking is nothing short of heaven! Chicken, simmered in coconut milk, garlic, fresh herbs and onions...I'm there for it!

2 pounds or 6-8 chicken pieces
1-2 tablespoons olive oil
Kosher salt
Ground black pepper
Seasoning salt
1 small yellow onion, diced
1 teaspoon fresh garlic, minced
3 teaspoons curry powder
1 teaspoon smoked paprika
1 can full fat coconut milk
1 1/2 cups organic chicken stock
2 -3 tablespoons fresh herbs (thyme, parsley)
2 medium carrots, chopped

Cooked brown rice

Season chicken pieces generously and set aside.

In a large stockpot, heat oil over medium heat, add chicken pieces and brown on both sides, approximately 2-3 minutes. Remove chicken.

Add more oil if needed. Add onions, garlic, curry powder and paprika to the stockpot and cook for 2-3 minutes, stirring frequently. Add the coconut milk and stock to the pot and stir.

Return chicken to the pan; along with herbs and carrots. Cover. Cook for about 45 minutes or until chicken is no longer pink and cooked through.

Serve over cooked brown rice.

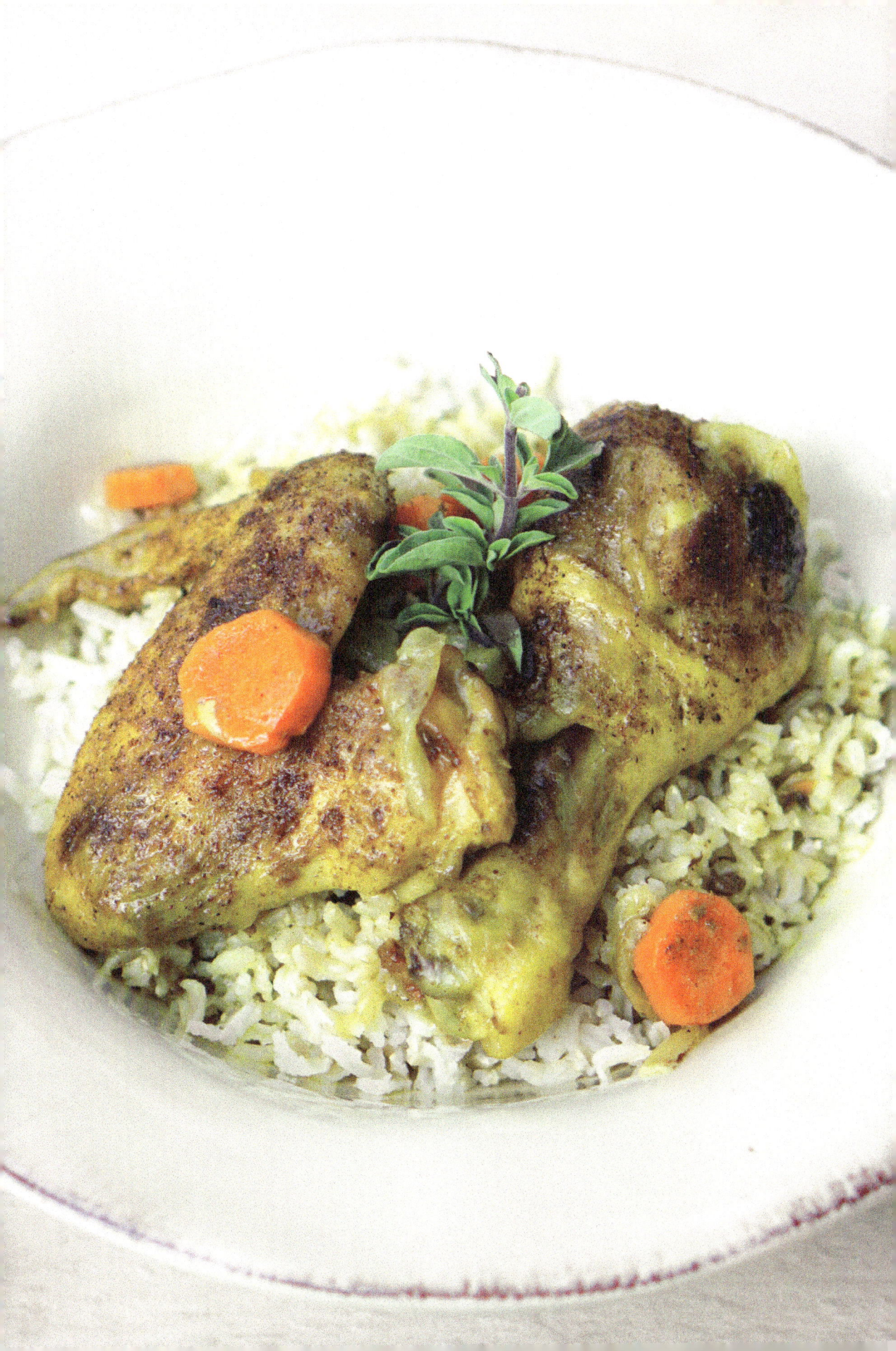

roasted orange chicken

[Serves 4]

Roasted chicken is the first dish I probably learned how to make. Just clean the chicken, season it and plop it in the oven. But now it does not have to taste like the first dish you ever made. Kick it up with this mix of orange and spices; a great Sunday meal or holiday favorite.

1 whole organic chicken
2 large oranges, cut into quarters
1 large yellow onion, roughly chopped
4 sprigs of fresh thyme
2 cloves garlic, peeled
1-2 tablespoons olive oil
Ground cumin
Seasoning salt
Kosher salt and ground black pepper
1 cup fresh squeezed orange juice or water

Pre-heat oven to 375 degrees.

Discard giblets and neck from chicken and clean chicken thoroughly. Pat dry.

Put half the onion, 2 sprigs thyme, and garlic cloves inside the cavity of the chicken. Tie the legs together with kitchen twine.

Place chicken in cast iron skillet or roasting pan. Drizzle some orange juice over the chicken. Rub chicken with olive oil. Season chicken with cumin, seasoning salt, kosher salt and ground black pepper. Add remaining onion and orange slices around chicken. Pour the liquid into the roasting pan.

Place in oven and roast, uncovered, for about 1.5 hours or until thermometer inserted into thickest part of thigh reads 165°. Baste when necessary.

Once removed, allow chicken to rest for at least ten minutes before carving.

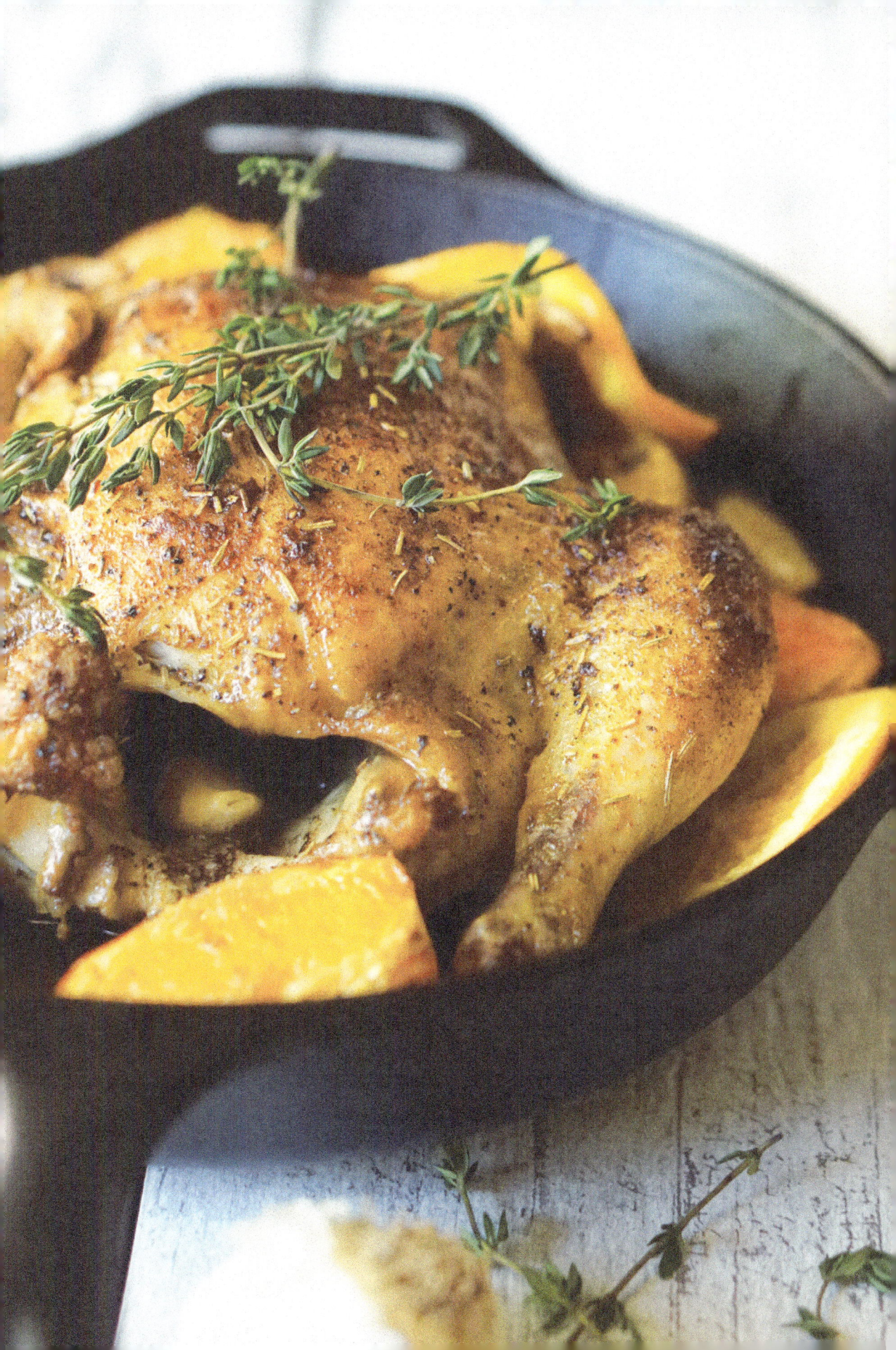

salmon

[Serves 2]

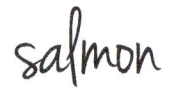

Salmon is one of my favorite foods to eat. I used to purchase my salmon without the skin but that is honestly the best part of the fish, in my opinion. It is packed with fatty acids so it has some health benefits too. Make your salmon with the crispy skin, just like they do at your favorite restaurant. Ready in 15 minutes or less!

2 fresh salmon filets
Olive oil
Kosher salt
Freshly cracked black pepper
1 tablespoon butter, room temperature

Clean the salmon and pat it dry.

Preheat the oven broiler to high.

Lightly coat the salmon with olive oil. If you are leaving the skin on, rub the softened butter into the skin of the salmon and place in the refrigerator for 15 minutes.

Remove the salmon from the fridge and season it with salt and black pepper.

Place the salmon on a broiler pan or cast iron skillet, skin side up, approximately 5 inches from the heat. Broil for 7-9 minutes in the oven. If the skin is getting too dark, move the fish a little further from the heat source.

Serve with your favorite veggies, over a bed of lentils, on a salad or with a salsa on top.

Salsa:

1/2 cup organic strawberries, diced
1/2 cup cucumber, diced
1/2 cup mangoes, diced
1/4 cup red onion, chopped
1 handful of fresh cilantro leaves (or parsley), washed and rough chopped
2 tablespoons fresh lime juice
Salt and pepper, to taste

.....
Do not serve the salmon with the skin side down once you have worked so hard to achieve the crispy outer skin. If you do, it will become soggy.

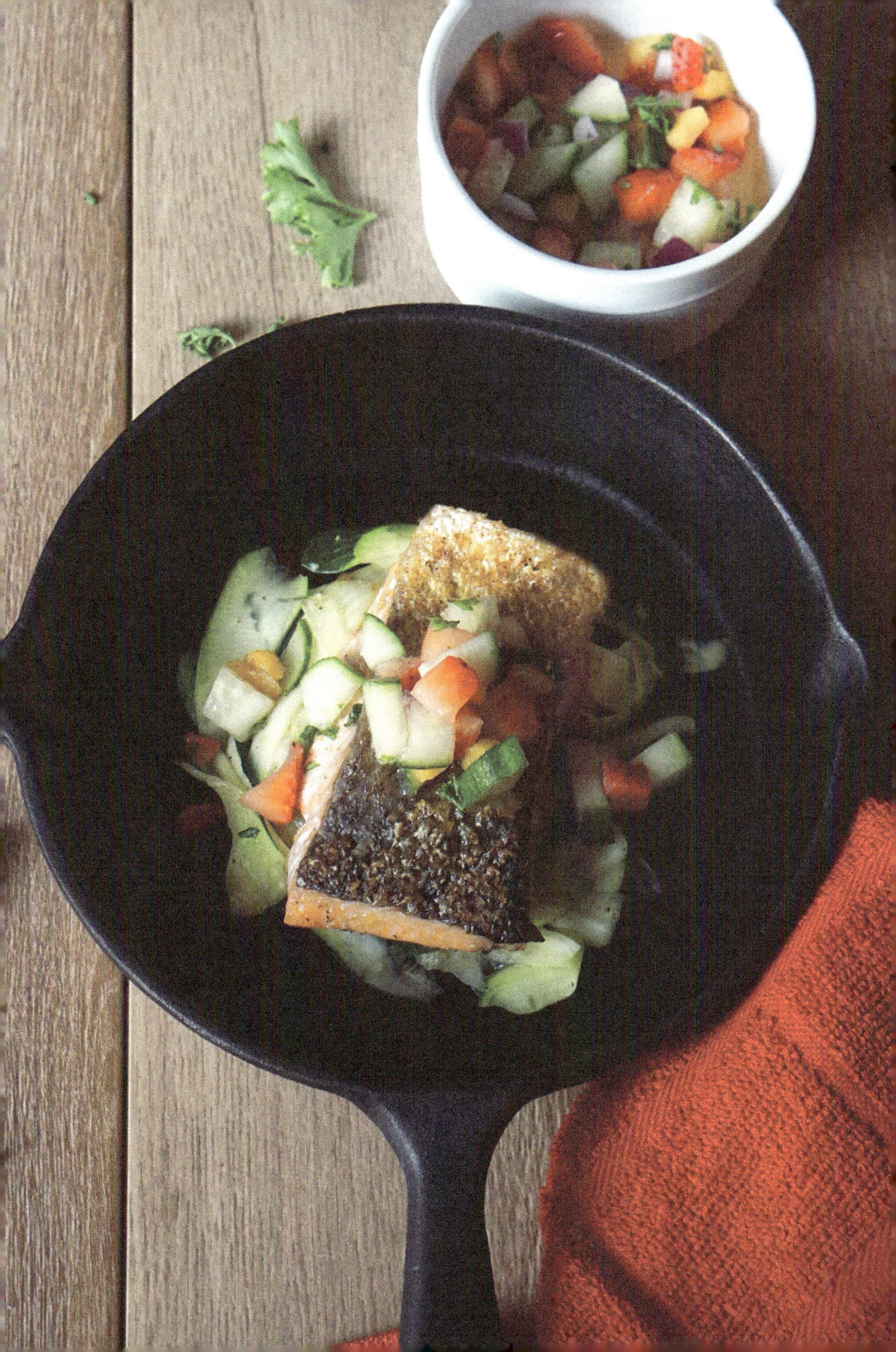

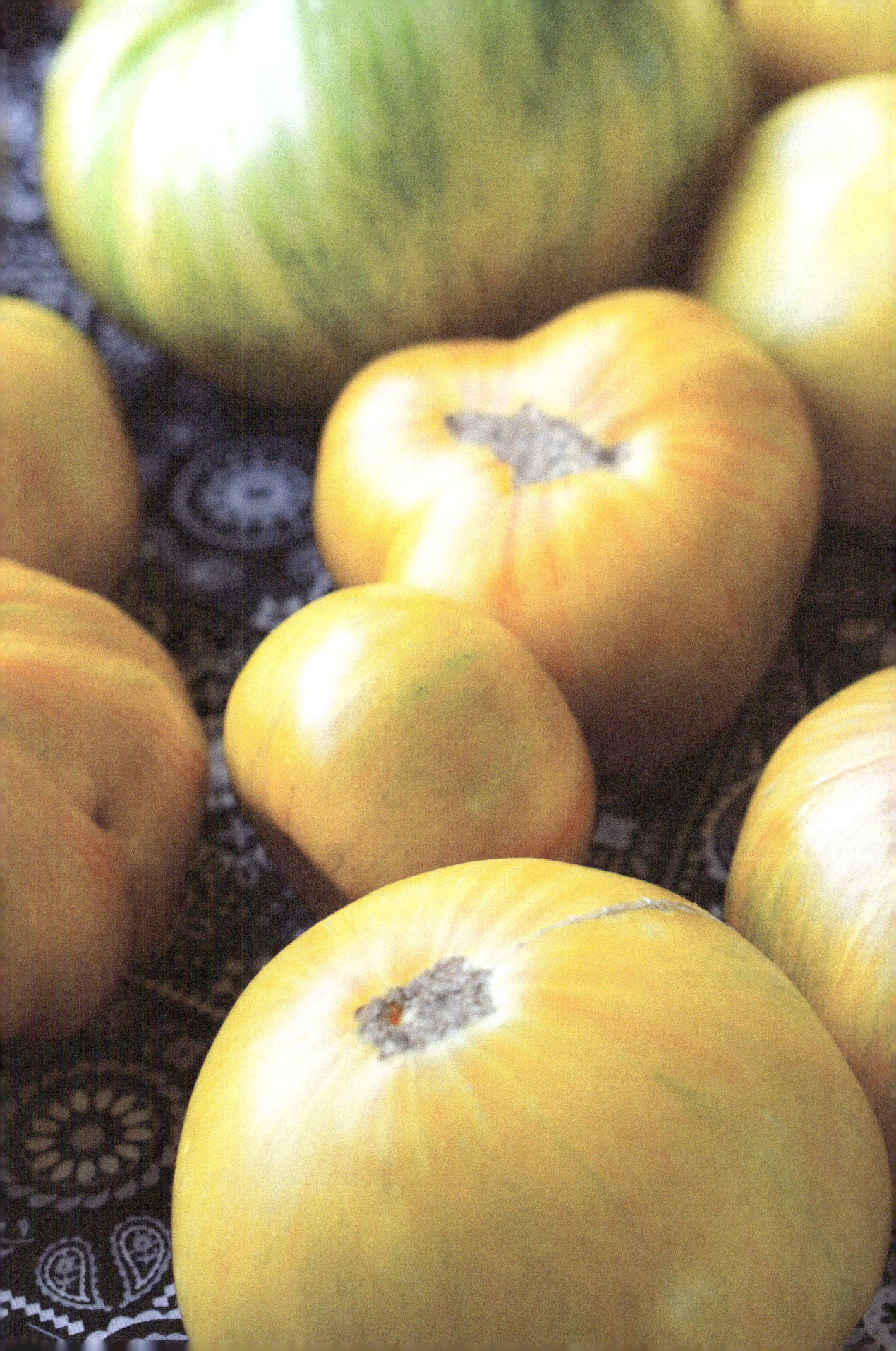

sides 'n such

89 **Roasted Brussels Sprouts**
These are not the Brussels sprouts your mama used to make you eat when you were younger.

91 **Sweet Potato Fries**
A healthy way to still enjoy fries.

92 **Braised Spinach and Kale Medley**
This quick and easy dish goes great alongside...well, almost anything.

94 **Roasted Carrots**
Roasted rainbow carrots are a great complement with roasted chicken. Savory and sweet!

96 **Applesauce**
Make homemade applesauce in 20 minutes or less. Great in breads, pancakes or all by its lonesome.

97 **Roasted Corn Salad**
This easy summer salad is hard to put down.

99 **Roasted Red Pepper Hummus**
A great dip for veggies or sauce for sandwiches. You'll never eat store bought again.

102 **Apple Chips**
You don't need a dehydrator to enjoy these delicious apple chips.

103 **Kale Chips**
The perfect low carb snack!

roasted brussels sprouts

[Serves 2]

I hated Brussels sprouts when I was younger. I am not sure if it was the way it was prepared or if it was just because it was a green vegetable and what kid wants to eat their green veggies? Either way, it was not something I was happy to see at the dinner table. Today, it is one of my favorites, raw or roasted, and is a staple in my kitchen.

1 pound Brussels sprouts, ends trimmed
Dash of lemon juice
2 tablespoons extra virgin olive oil
1/2 teaspoon Kosher salt
1/4 teaspoon freshly ground black pepper

Turkey bacon, *optional*

Clean the Brussels sprouts and trim the ends.

Preheat cast iron pan or baking sheet in oven at 400 for about ten minutes.

Toss the Brussels sprouts in lemon juice, olive oil and salt and pepper until coated.

Arrange in pan in a single layer and roast until golden brown, about 30-35 minutes.

Sprinkle with turkey bacon, if desired.

.....
Brussels sprouts are a part of the cruciferous family and have cancer prevention properties, particularly if eaten raw. Adding them to your diet is a great benefit to your health!

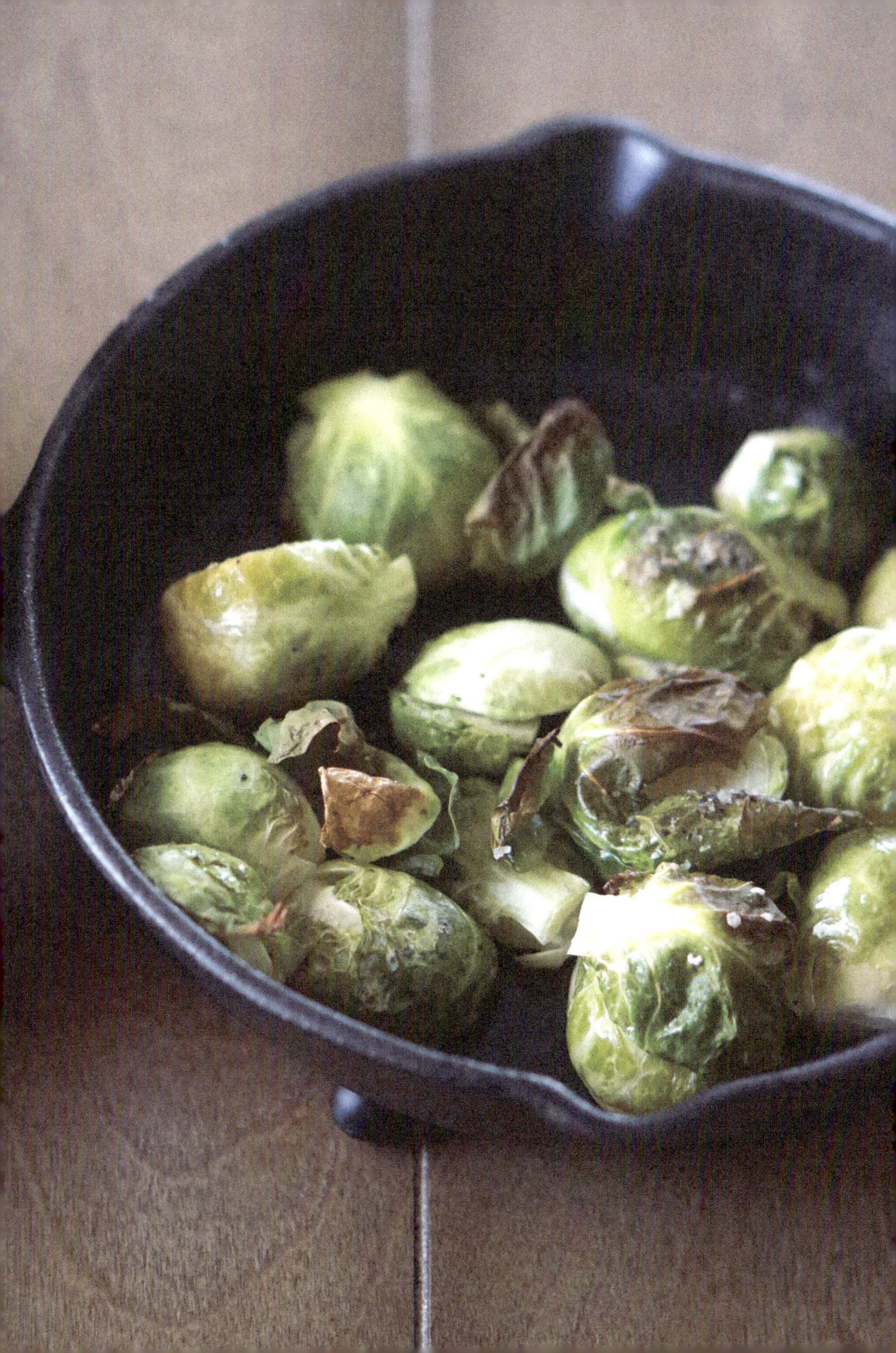

sweet potato fries

[Serves 1-2]

I eat sweet potatoes almost every day! Since I do not consume sugar, unless in the natural form, sweet potatoes serve as my dessert on most evenings. That said, one of my favorite sides is sweet potato fries. The smoked paprika gives them a little kick. Simply delicious!

2 pounds organic sweet potatoes, scrubbed
2 tablespoons olive oil or virgin coconut oil
1 teaspoon kosher salt
1 teaspoon smoked paprika
1/2 teaspoon freshly ground black pepper
1 teaspoon garlic powder, *optional*

Preheat oven to 400 degrees F.

Leave the skin on and cut sweet potatoes into thin fries, as evenly as possible.

Place in large bowl and drizzle with oil. Mixed seasonings together in a small bowl. Sprinkle fries with seasonings and toss until coated.

Transfer fries to large baking sheets and arrange in a single layer. Bake for 15 minutes and turn to other side. Bake for 10 to 15 minutes more, or until crispy.

Remove from oven and serve hot.

.....
If you deal with a lot of inflammation in your body, you do not want to consume sweet potatoes or other nightshades on a regular basis.

braised spinach and kale medley

[Serves 2]

Braising is the process of simmering food in a small amount of liquid in a covered or uncovered pan or casserole. This medley is a great accompaniment for a fried or poached egg, but is the perfect side to almost any dish. Best eaten the same day.

2 tablespoons olive oil
1/2 small yellow onion
2 cups fresh kale
2 cups fresh spinach
1 cup shiitake mushrooms
Kosher salt, to taste
Freshly ground black pepper, to taste
Dash of paprika
1/2 to 1 teaspoon crushed red pepper flakes
1/4 cup organic chicken stock
1 teaspoon of organic apple cider vinegar

Clean kale and spinach thoroughly and rough chop it.

Add olive oil to large saute pan over medium heat. Add the onions and mushrooms and cook until onions are translucent, about 3-5 minutes. Add greens; sprinkle with salt, pepper, paprika and red pepper flakes.

Add chicken stock and vinegar, cover and cook just until wilted. Serve immediately.

.....

If you are not a fan of kale's bitter taste, try eating red kale, which is not quite as bitter.

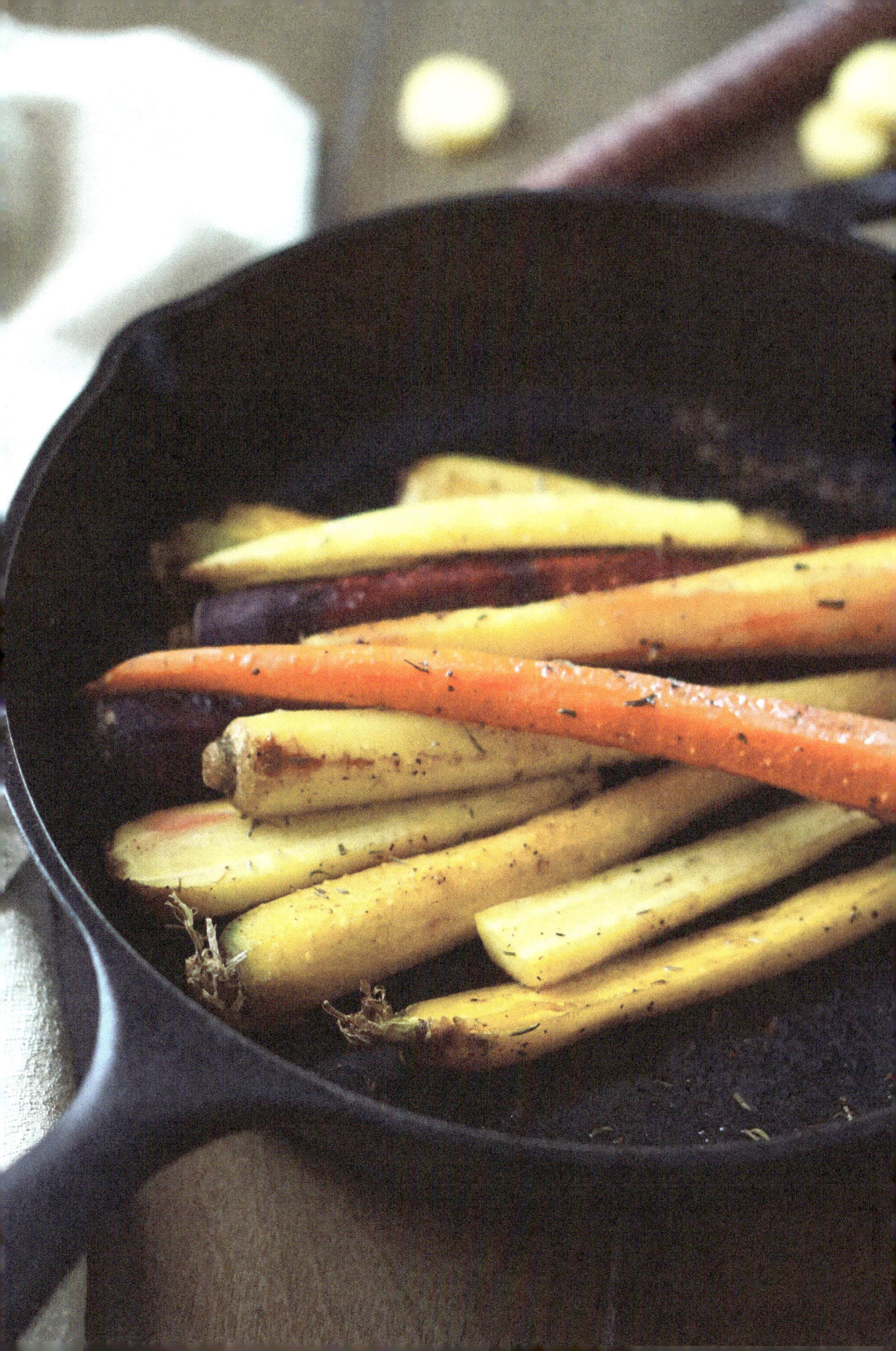

roasted carrots

[Serves 4]

Impress your guests with this simple, colorful, savory dish that is full of flavor. These carrots are great for a Sunday or holiday dinner and I particularly love them with poultry dishes.

1 bag of rainbow carrots
2 tablespoons virgin coconut oil
1/3 cup freshly squeezed orange juice
2 teaspoons of savory
Kosher salt and pepper, to taste
1/2 teaspoon of cumin
1 teaspoon of nutmeg
1 teaspoon of ginger

Preheat oven to 425 degrees.

Clean carrots and pat them dry.

In a large bowl, toss carrots in coconut oil, orange juice, and seasonings. Arrange on a baking sheet in a single layer.

Roast for 30 minutes, turning once, or until tender and caramelized.

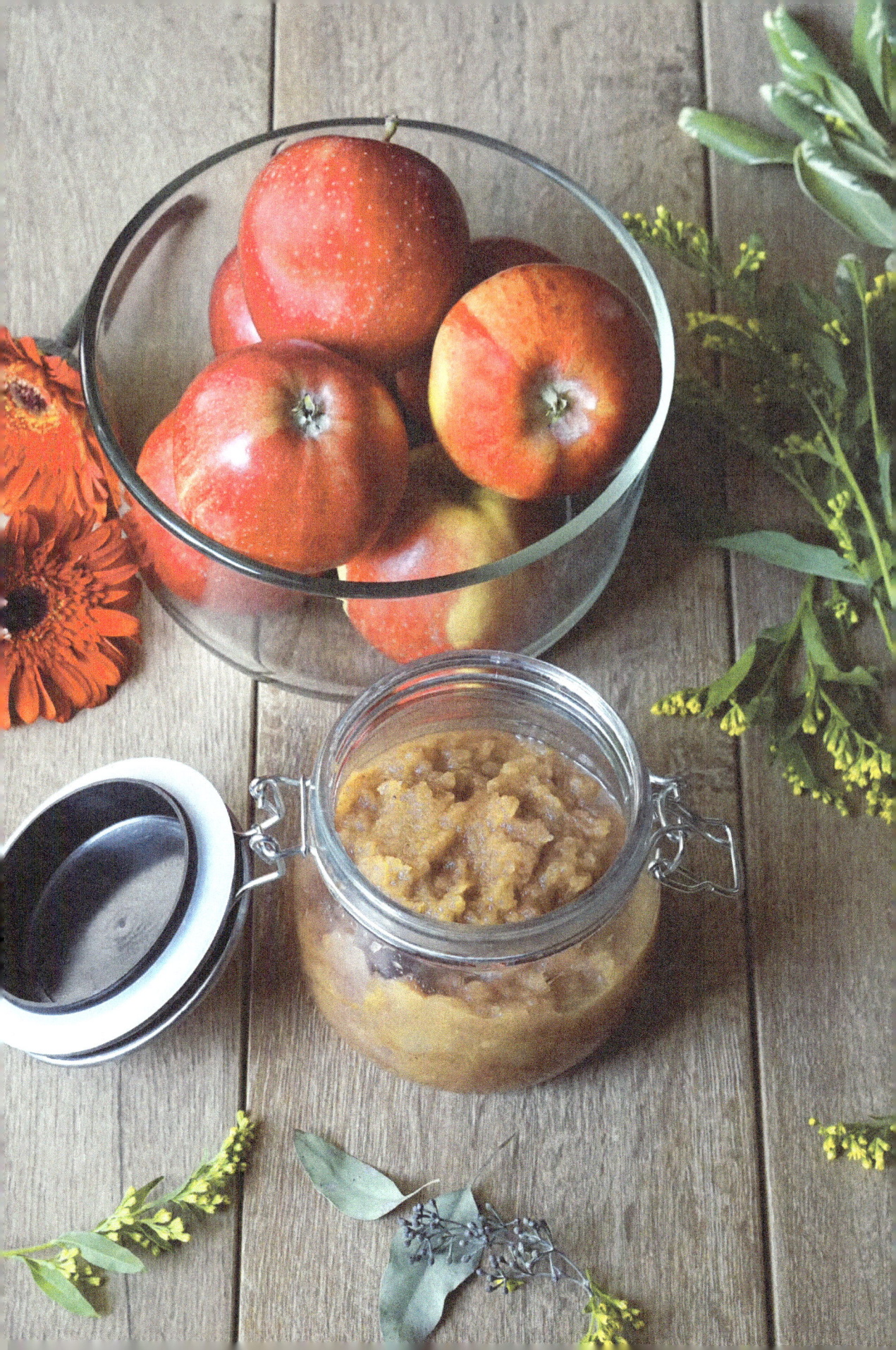

chunky applesauce

[Serves 2]

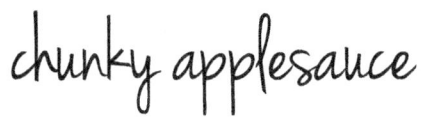

You will never buy store-bought applesauce again once you realize how simple it is to make your own at home. Hearty and pleasing by itself or it can be used in pancakes, cakes or muffins to yield a moist, delicious baked good.

4 large apples
Dash of lemon juice
3/4 cup water
1/2 teaspoon ground cinnamon
A pinch of nutmeg

Wash, peel, core and chop apples. Cut apples into chunks.

In a medium saucepan, combine apples, lemon juice and water. Cover and bring to a light boil. Reduce heat to medium low and simmer for approximately 15 minutes. (Add more water if necessary).

Add cinnamon and nutmeg and continue to cook for another 10-15 minutes. Once the mixture has softened, mash the apples until desired consistency is achieved.

If you want to eliminate the chunks completely, use an immersion blender, or mini food processor, for a smoother consistency.

.....

If you want to add layers of flavor to your applesauce, use a variety of apples. Some of the recommended ones are Fuji, Braeburn, Rome, McIntosh, Golden Delicious, and Gala. Combinations of these will give you a combination of sweet and tart.

roasted corn salad

[Serves 4]

Nothing says summer like fresh, sweet corn on the cob, well...except ice cream. Need a quick dish to take to a cookout? This corn salad is a sure winner. It is very versatile as well. You can add onion, red pepper, jalapeno...whatever your tastebuds desire. Great as a side dish on its own or as a salsa for salmon, chicken breasts or steak.

5 ears of corn
1 medium green pepper (or jalapeno), diced
1/2 cup red onion, diced (optional)
1/2 cup chopped fresh parsley or cilantro
2 tablespoons freshly squeezed lime juice
1/4 cup extra virgin olive oil
Salt and pepper, to taste

Preheat oven to 425 degrees.

Rub a little olive oil on corn and wrap in foil. Roast the ears of corn on a cookie sheet for about 20 minutes. Allow corn to cool. Remove the kernels and place in a large bowl.

Add the green pepper, onion, parsley or cilantro and toss. Add the juice from the limes and the olive oil and combine. Add salt and pepper, to taste.

Cool in the fridge and serve.

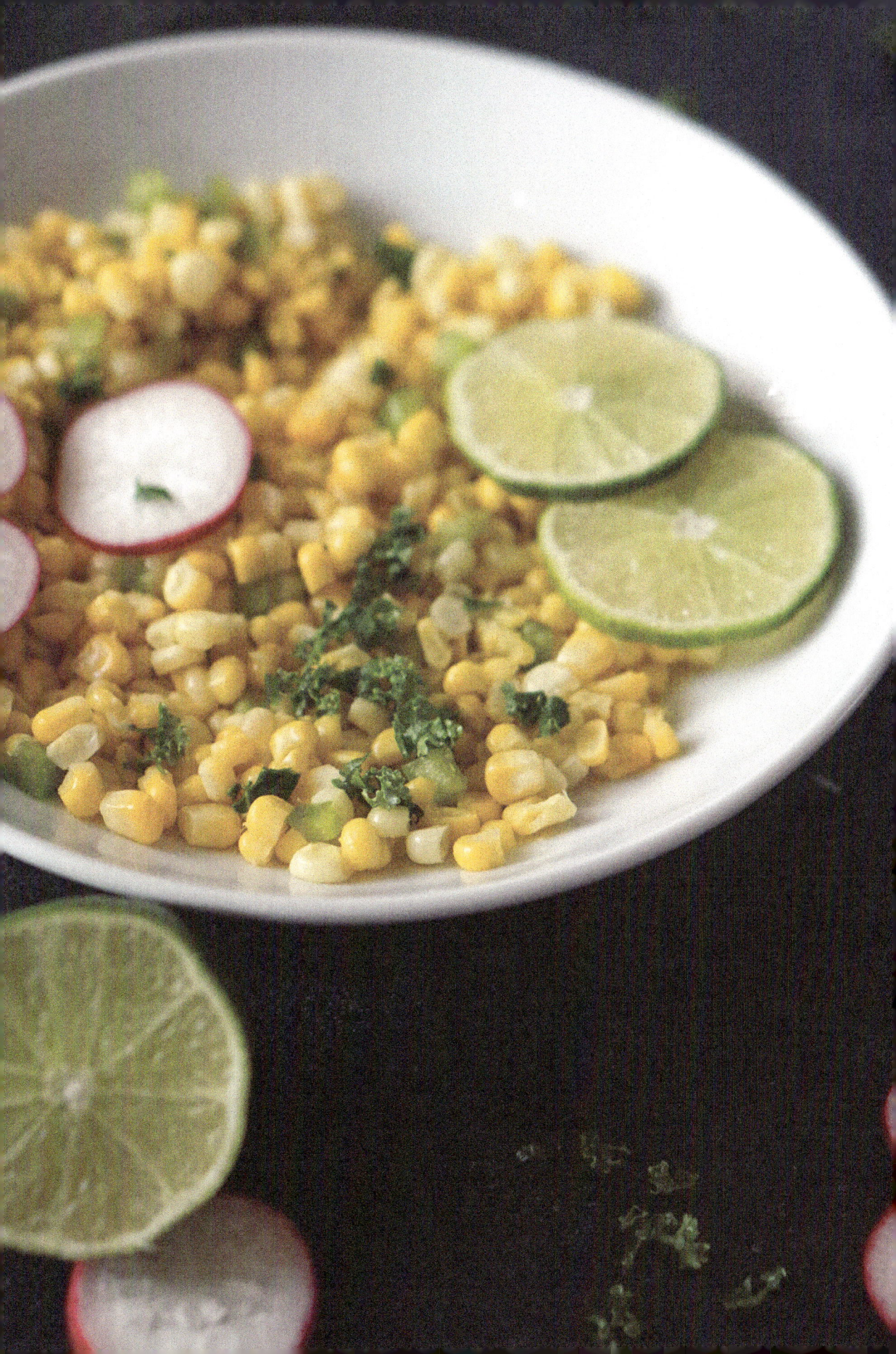

roasted red pepper hummus

[Serves 4]

Hummus is a thick spread made from ground chickpeas, olive oil, lemon juice, and garlic, made originally in the Middle East. There are so many different varieties - pumpkin, garlic, black bean, sun dried tomato and spinach hummus, to name a few. I eat this on burgers, with raw vegetables, on naan and use it as the sauce for homemade pizza.

15 oz can of chickpeas (or garbanzo beans)
1 teaspoon paprika
Pinch of cayenne pepper
1/2 teaspoon cumin
1-2 roasted red peppers
2 garlic cloves
2 tablespoon raw tahini, *optional*
1 tablespoon lemon juice
Salt and pepper, to taste
1/4 cup extra virgin olive oil

To roast red peppers:

Wash the pepper thoroughly.
Preheat oven to 450 degrees.
Line a baking sheet with foil.
Arrange peppers on baking sheet, spaced apart.
Roast for 30 minutes, turning once.
Place peppers in a glass dish and cover.
Peel the skin, remove the seeds and pepper is ready for use in your favorite dish.

To make the hummus:

Drain the garbanzo beans; preserve the liquid. Blend the garbanzo beans in a good processor. Add remaining ingredients, except for the olive oil and puree. Slowly add in olive oil until smooth. If hummus is too thick, add some of the liquid from the garbanzo beans, a teaspoon at a time. Chill and set for approximately an hour. Garnish and serve.

.....
You can cheat and purchase the roasted red bell peppers in
the jar for this quick and easy hummus dish.
But it is just as easy to roast them on your own.

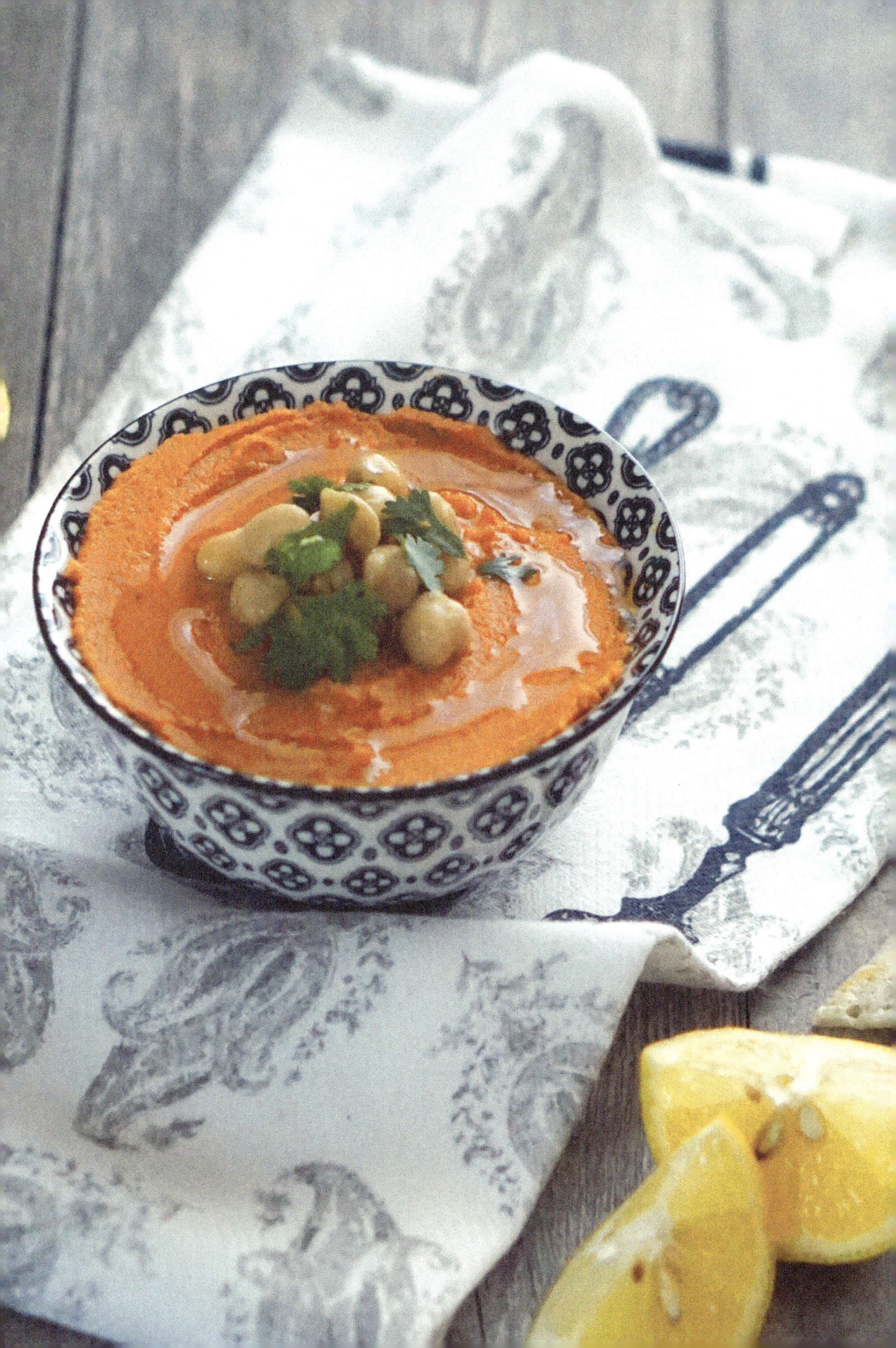

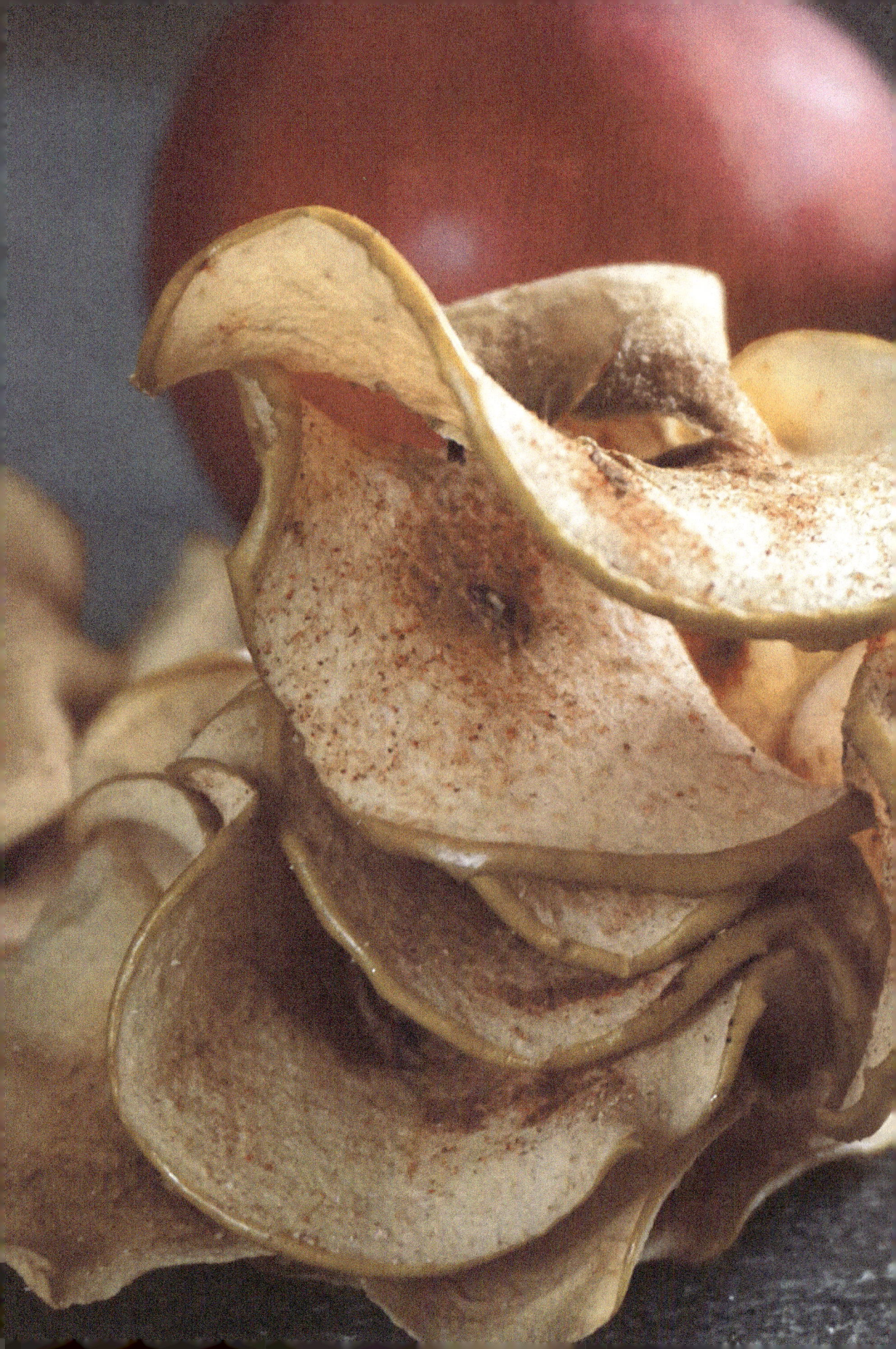

apple chips

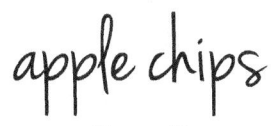

[Serves 1]

My first experience with apple chips came shortly after one of my favorite lunch spots added a salad to their menu with apple chips as the garnish. I became obsessed with them and started ordering them by the case. And then I realized I was wasting money on something I could easily make at home. So I started making them myself. They take a bit of time to make but definitely worth the wait. Dehydrator not necessary! Patience is.

2 large apples (Red Delicious or Granny Smith)
2-3 teaspoons of stevia in the raw
1 teaspoon cinnamon

Preheat oven to 200 degrees.

Use mandolin to thinly slice apples. Arrange apples in a single layer on a cookie sheet lined with parchment paper.

Combine stevia and cinnamon in a small bowl. Using a sieve, sprinkle over apple slices.

Bake in bottom part of oven until apples are crispy and dry, about 2 hours. Every 30 minutes flip the apple slices over to ensure they bake evenly. Once chips are done, let them cool completely.

Best eaten the same day.

kale chips

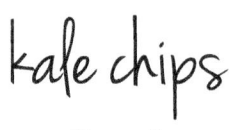

[Serves 1]

Kale chips are a light, airy, low-carb snack that takes minutes to make and is great when you can't have regular chips but crave something crunchy.

1 medium bunch kale
Olive oil spray
Kosher salt
Sesame seeds, optional

Preheat oven to 300 degrees.

Wash kale leaves thoroughly and dry completely.

Cut the ribs out of the kale leaves and discard them. Trim leaves into small sections.

Lightly spray kale with olive oil. Sprinkle kale with kosher salt. Lay in a single layer on a baking sheet.

Bake for 10-12 minutes, or until crispy, keeping an eye out because the leaves brown quickly.

Remove from oven and cool. Kale chips will crisp up more as they cool. Serve immediately.

.....

Kale chips can be bitter if you use Lacinato kale. Use curly kale if you prefer less of a bite.

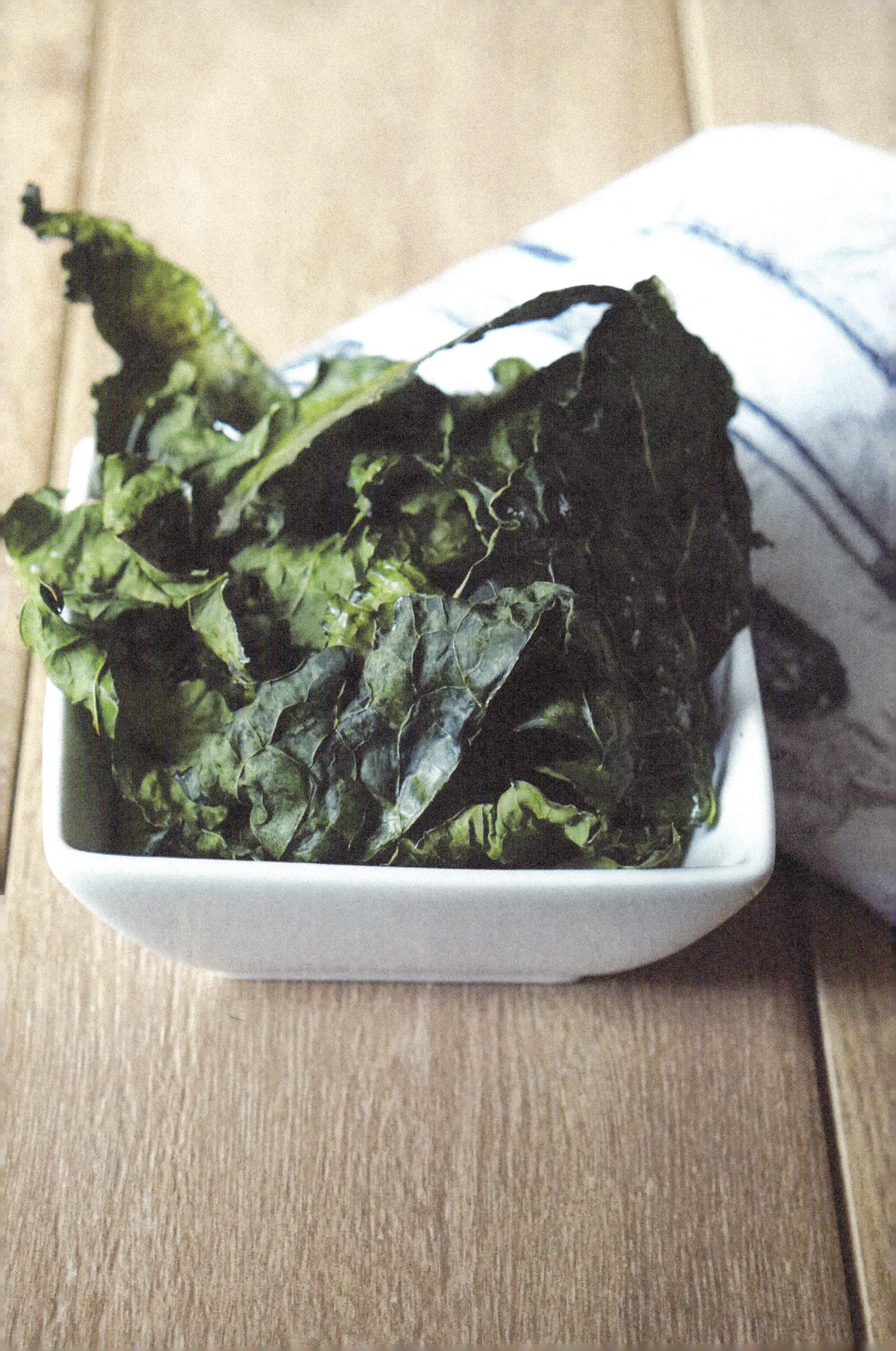

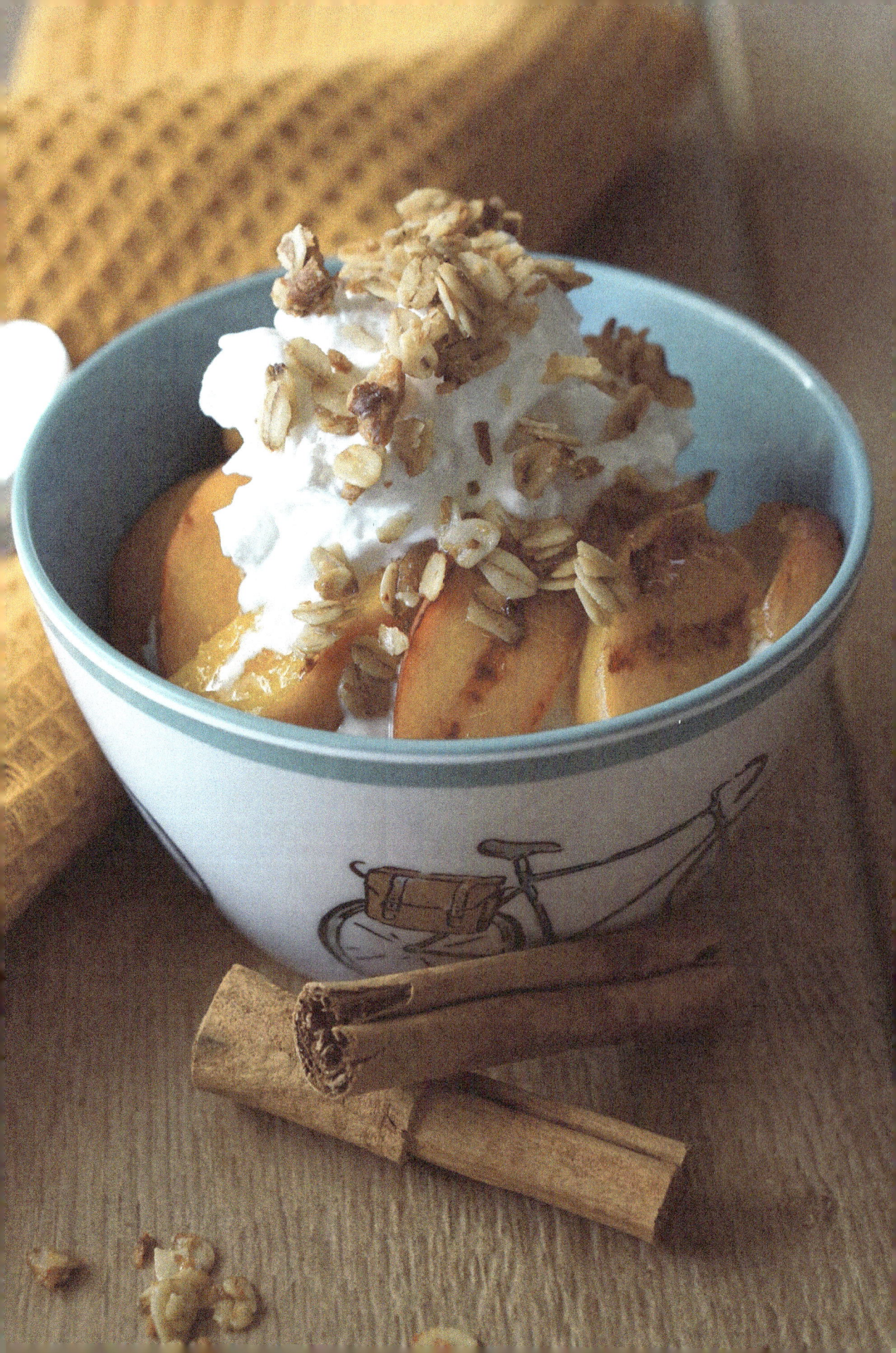

desserts

108 **Avocado Tart**
Not quite key lime pie but pretty tangy and rich and delicious. A great summer dessert.

110 **Sorbet**
Berry and mango sorbet are two really simple, straight out of the blender recipes, that are great palate cleansers.

112 **Dairy-Free Ice cream**
Soon as you thought you could never eat ice cream again...there is a dairy-free, sugar-free version that will make you fall in love with dessert all over again.

113 **Sweet Potato Bread**
This bread is simply delicious. Great alongside a cup of chamomile honey tea. Pair it with a whipped orange cinnamon butter and curl up under your favorite blanket.

115 **Lemon Pound Cake**
This bright cake is a great finish to any dinner. Well, it is great for breakfast or snack too. Sssshhh....if you don't tell, I won't tell!

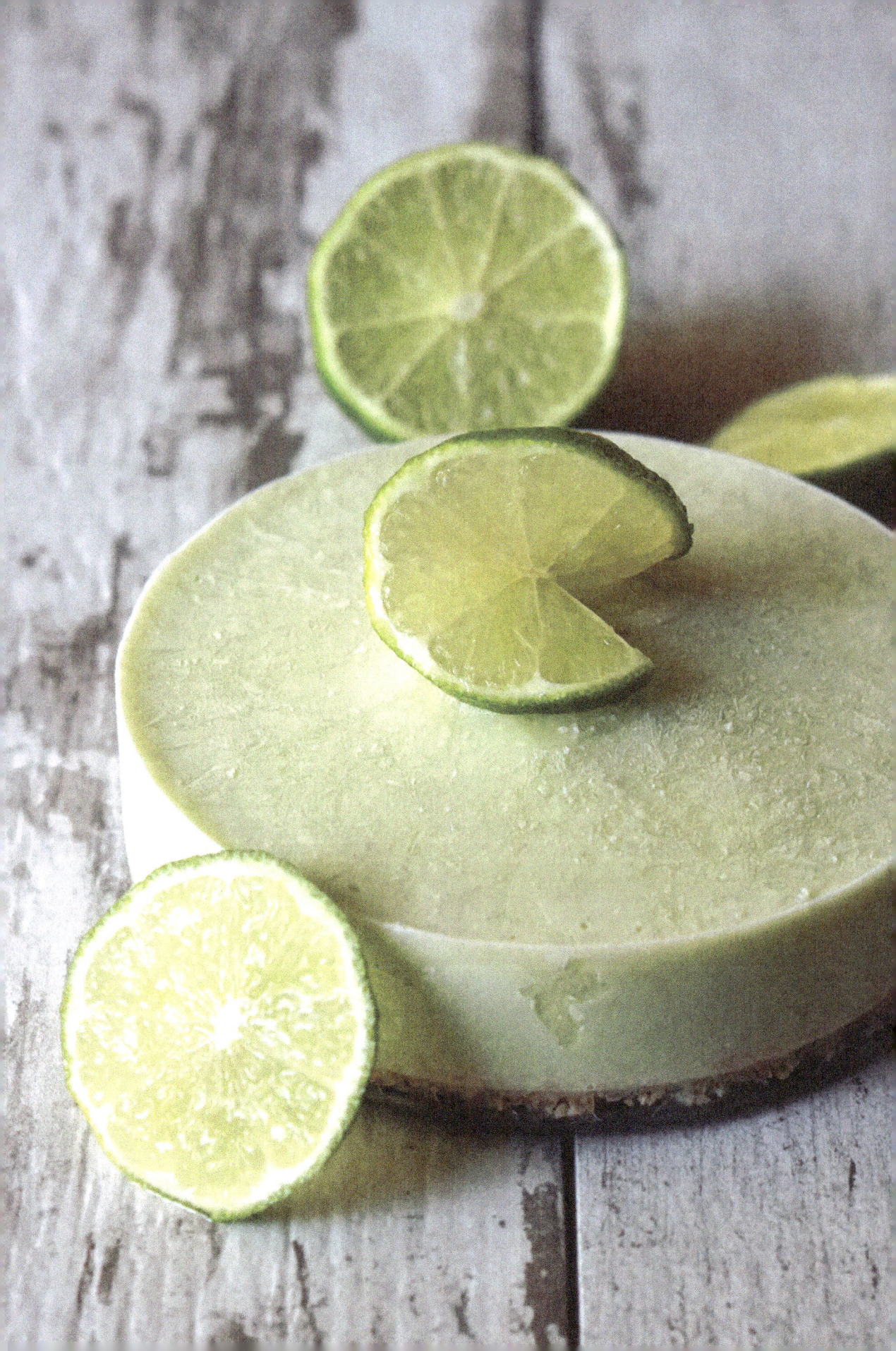

avocado tart

[Serves 2]

This is a frozen dessert so I love to eat it in the warmer months. It is tart, coconutty and is a great after dinner dessert. Add some toasted coconut flakes to give it some added texture.

Crust:
3/4 cup almonds
1/2 cup unsweetened coconut flakes
3 teaspoons coconut oil, melted
1 dropper liquid stevia

Tart:
2 avocados
Juice of one lime
1/2 cup full-fat coconut milk
Lime zest
1 teaspoon coconut oil, melted
2 droppers liquid stevia

For the crust:
Blend together the ingredients in a food processor until moist and sticky. Press into bottom of mini-springform pan.

For the filling:
Place tart ingredients in food processor or blender. Process until blended. Pour into springform pan, smoothing the top with a spoon. Place tart in the freezer until frozen (2-4 hours).

Once frozen, remove tart from springform pan with a knife. Let thaw for 10 minutes before serving. Garnish with lime zest, toasted coconut or lime wedge.

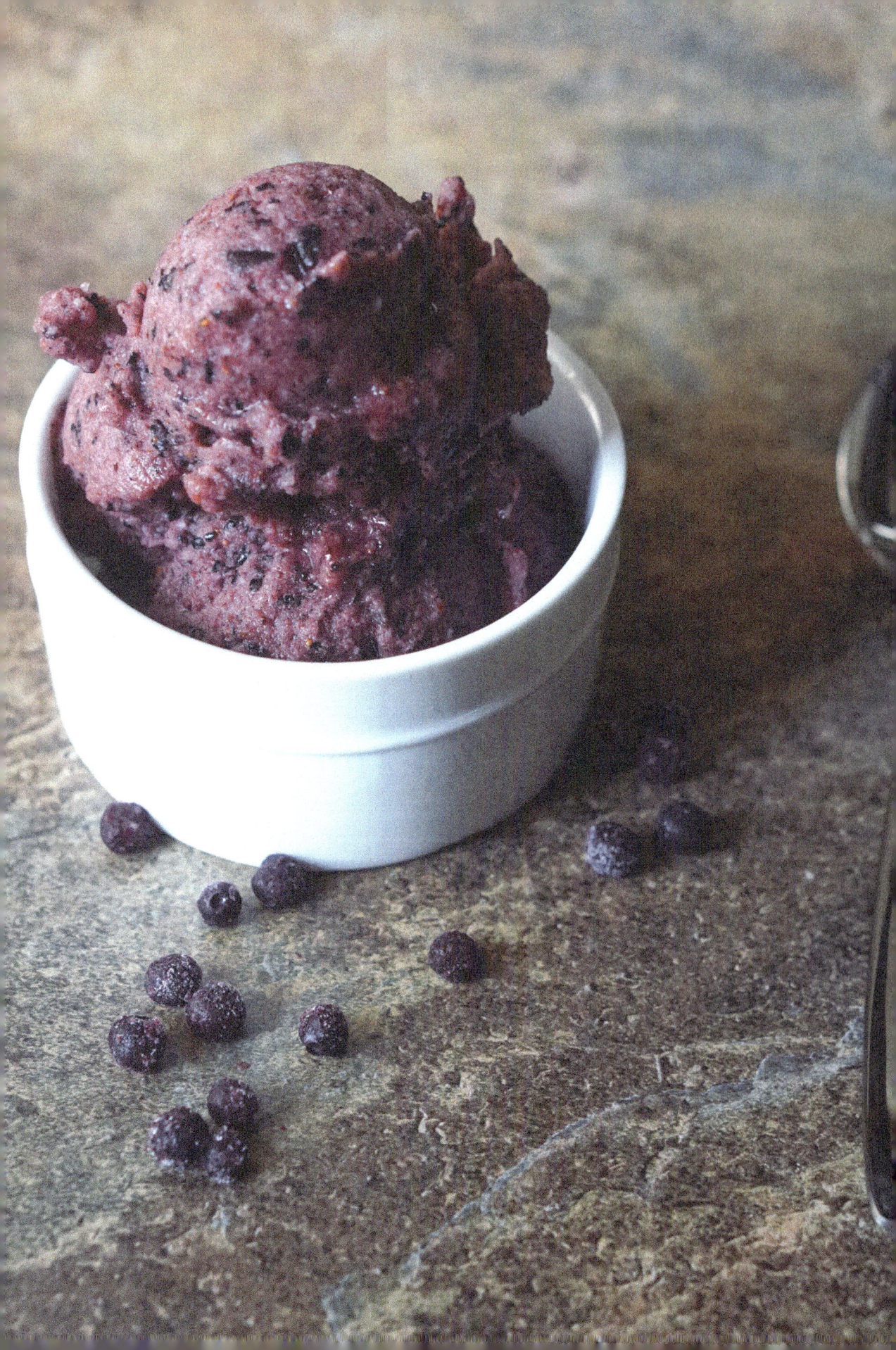

sorbet

[Serves 2]

Nothing like a big bowl of ice cream on a blazing hot, summer day! These sorbet recipes are made in the blender so they are ready in minutes.

Berry Sorbet:

4 cups frozen mixed berries
1 can full fat coconut milk
3 droppers of liquid stevia

Mango Sorbet:

2 cups frozen mango chunks
1/2 cup coconut milk
Dash of lime juice
1 dropper of liquid stevia

Process ingredients in high powered blender until creamy.

If you like soft serve consistency, you can serve immediately after processing. If not, freeze for 2 hours. Take out to soften 10 minutes before serving. No ice cream maker needed.

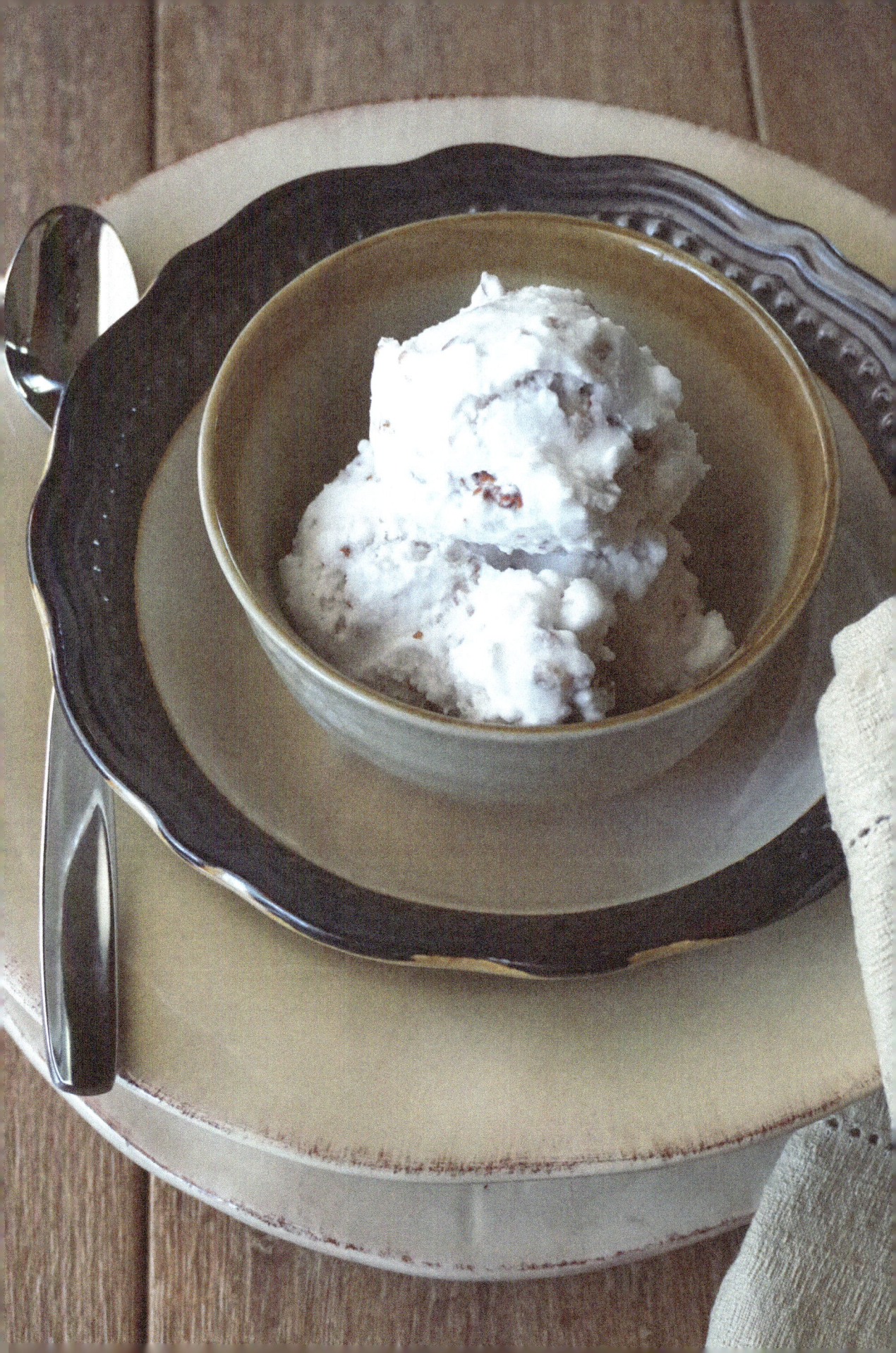

dairy-free ice cream

[Serves 1-2]

Since I used to be a baker, one of the things I disliked most about my lifestyle change was the lack of dessert in my diet. Initially I ate almonds and apples for dessert nightly and that was just not going to cut it. These dairy-free ice creams are so rich and creamy. You will have trouble believing that they are actually not bad for you.

Vanilla Ice Cream (Food Processor):

1 can full fat coconut milk
3 droppers liquid stevia (or 3 tablespoons raw honey)

For the vanilla ice cream:
Whisk full fat coconut milk with stevia. Freeze the coconut milk overnight on a cookie sheet, covered with parchment paper. (If you do not use the parchment paper, you will not be able to get it off of the baking sheet). Break the pieces up once it is frozen and process in a food processor until smooth. Serve.

Vanilla Ice Cream (Ice Cream Machine):

1 cup unsweetened almond milk
1 can coconut milk, full fat version
1 can coconut cream
Vanilla bean, optional
1/2 teaspoon tapioca starch or guar gum
3 droppers liquid stevia (or 3 tablespoons raw honey)

For the vanilla ice cream - Using ice cream maker:
Combine ingredients and place in refrigerator overnight to cool. Process in ice cream maker for 25 minutes. Place in freezer for 2 hours. Serve.

Butter Pecan Ice Cream:

1 can full fat unsweetened coconut milk
1 cup unsweetened almond milk
1/2 teaspoon alcohol-free vanilla extract
1 egg yolk
2 tablespoons arrowroot powder
3 droppers liquid stevia (or 3 tablespoons raw honey)
2 tablespoons unsalted butter
1 cup pecans
Himalayan sea salt

For the butter pecan ice cream:
Combine the milk, egg yolk, arrowroot powder, sweetener and salt in a saucepan and slowly bring the mixture to a light boil. Cool and then mix in the vanilla extract. Refrigerate overnight.

Melt butter in pan and add pecans.
Coat pecans in butter and salt them.
Roast for 5 minutes. Set aside and cool. Fold into ice cream mixture.

Process in ice cream maker for 25 minutes. Place in freezer for 2 hours. Serve.

.....

Because there is not as much fat content, this ice cream will get very hard. So take it out 15-20 minutes prior to serving each time. Add a teaspoon of xanthan gum or tapioca starch to get a creamier base.

sweet potato bread

[Serves 4-6]

Hello autumn! This sweet potato bread is amazing. I make some compound butter to go along with it - a bit of fresh orange juice, softened butter, cinnamon, and stevia and whip it with the stand mixer...and then add a cup of chamomile honey tea along with it. You won't want to put it down.

1 cup almond flour
1/4 cup coconut flour
1/2 teaspoon sea salt
1/2 teaspoon baking soda
1 1/2 teaspoon cinnamon
1 teaspoon nutmeg
1/2 cup sweet potato, cooked
1/2 teaspoon fresh orange zest
1/2 cup stevia in the raw
1/4 cup coconut oil
3 eggs
1/2 cup chopped walnuts, chopped

Preheat the oven to 350 degrees.

Combine the wet ingredients in a bowl, along with the sweet potato and orange zest.

Combine the dry ingredients in a separate bowl.

Mix the wet and dry ingredients together until incorporated.

Pour into loaf pan, lined with parchment paper, and bake for 50-60 minutes, or until toothpick comes out clean when inserted in the middle.

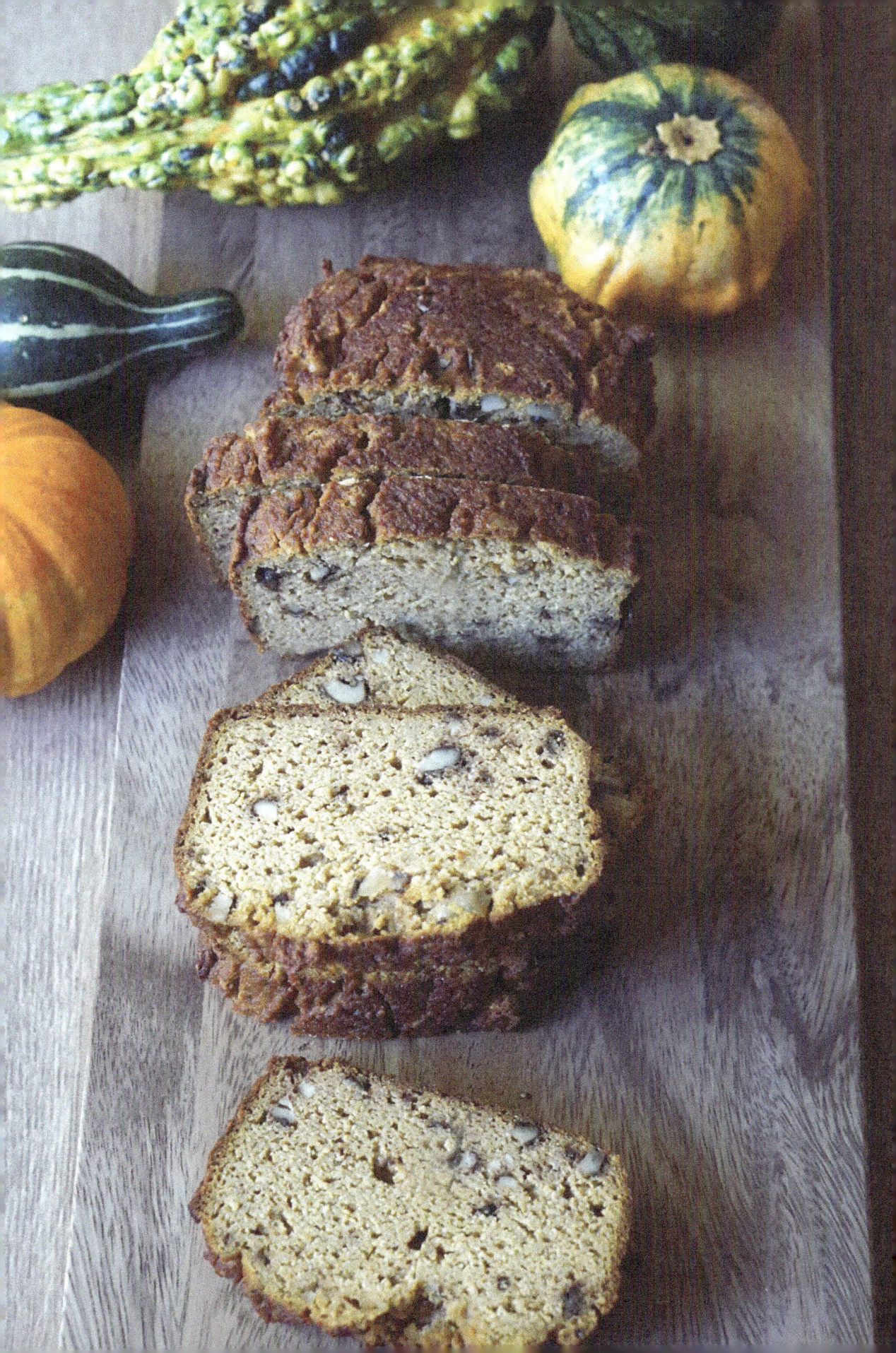

lemon pound cake

[Serves 4-6]

I had four favorite desserts before I started my clean eating journey - peach cobbler, key lime pie, cheesecake and pound cake. I am happy to have pound cake back in my diet on occasion. This is a really light, flavorful pound cake that can be eaten with coconut ice cream or by itself. Trust me, it won't be around the house for long.

2 cups Trader Joe's All Purpose GF Flour
4 teaspoons baking powder
1/2 teaspoon sea salt
1 1/2 cup stevia in the raw
1/2 cup coconut oil, melted
Juice of one large organic lemon
1 teaspoon alcohol-free vanilla extract
4 eggs, room temperature

Glaze *(Optional)*:
2 tablespoons coconut oil
1 dropper of liquid stevia
2 tablespoons full fat coconut milk
Dash of lemon juice

Preheat oven to 350 degrees.

Line a loaf pan with parchment paper (or you can grease and flour a small bundt pan).

Combine the flour, baking powder, salt and stevia.

In a separate bowl, combine the coconut oil, lemon juice, flavoring (vanilla extract) and eggs. Slowly incorporate the dry ingredients, mixing well.

Pour into loaf pan and bake for 50-60 minutes or until toothpick inserted in middle comes out clean. Remove from oven and let cool in pan for 10 minutes. Remove from loaf pan and allow to fully cool on a rack.

For the glaze:
Mix the ingredients together in a small saucepan. Remove from heat and set aside. Once the pound cake is done and slightly cooled, pour the glaze over the loaf.

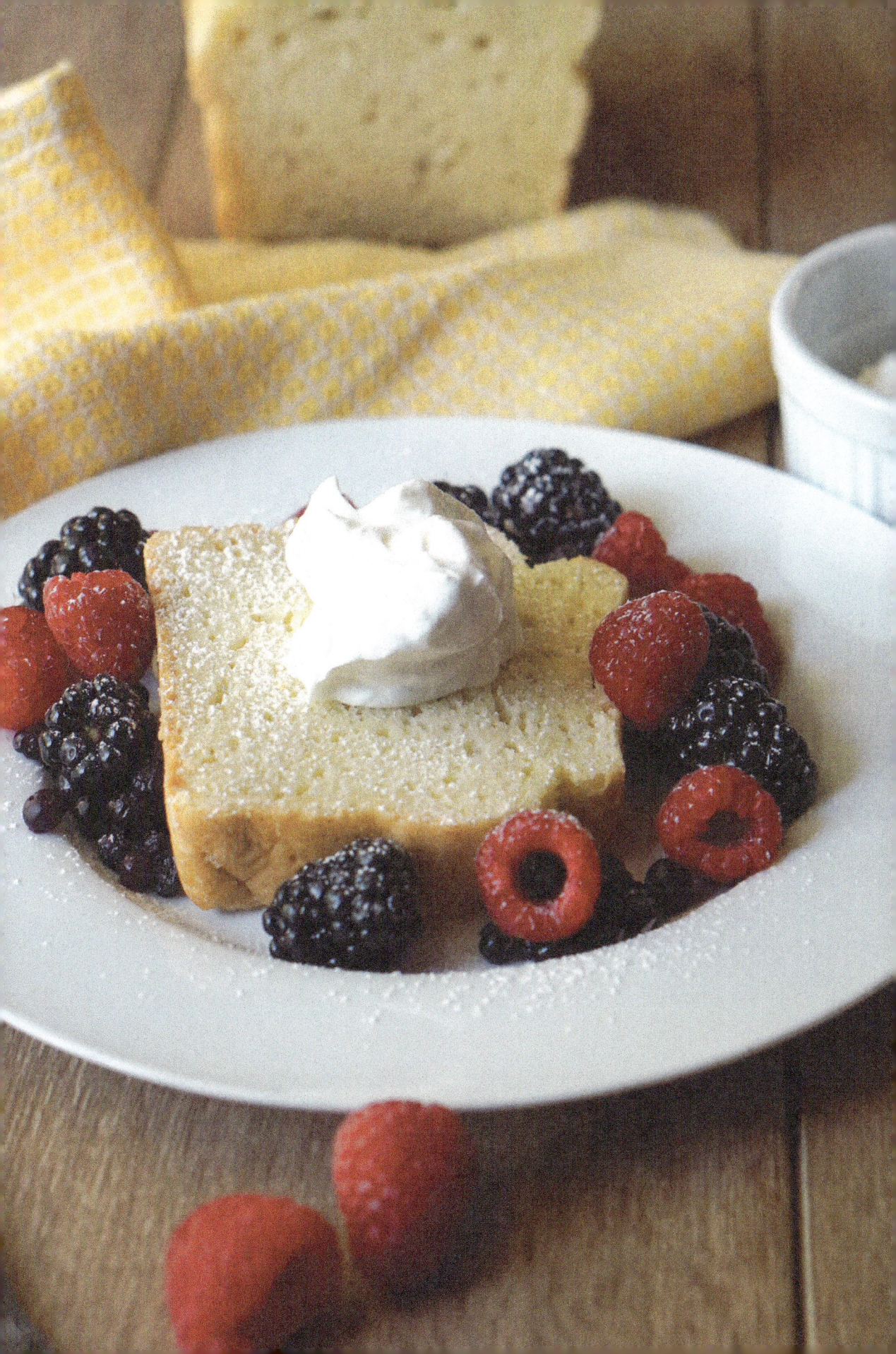

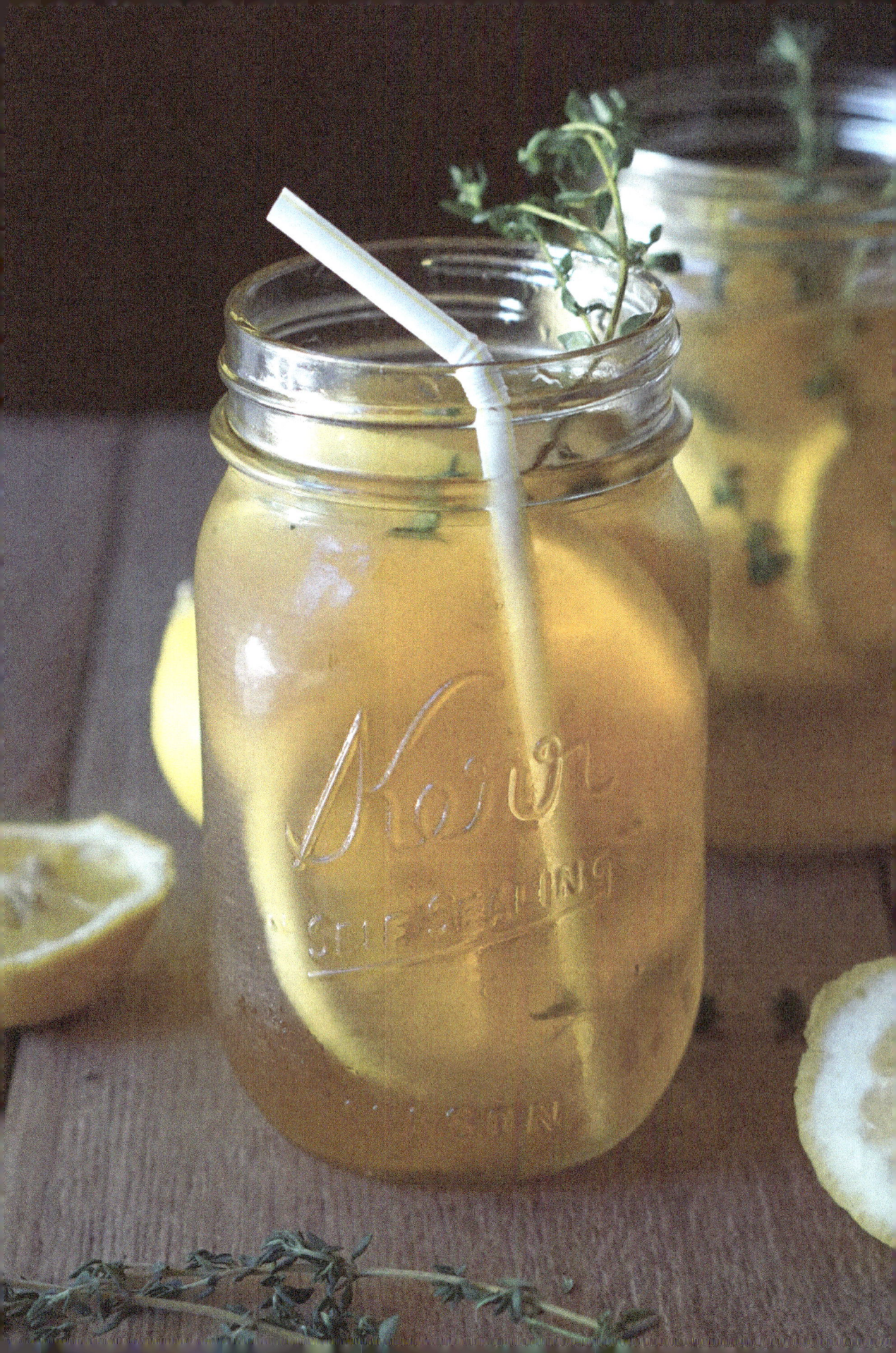

beverages

119 **Beet Juice**
Cleanse your liver and enjoy a sweet, tasty concoction at the same time!

121 **Carrot Juice**
This is a sweet and spicy, bright juice to get you started on your day.

123 **Green Drinks**
Boost your energy, get clearer skin, improve your waistline and help your digestive system with these green drinks.

127 **Turmeric Tea**
Hot or cold, reduce inflammation in your body with these two versions of turmeric tea.

130 **Healthy Mojito**
Ok, ok. This is really nothing more than a detox drink but it looks and sounds so inviting, it will make you want to infuse your water too!

132 **Immune Boosting Drinks**
Feel a cold or flu bug coming on? These immune boosting drinks will help get your body fight those invaders.

beet juice

[Serves 1]

You could not pay me to eat beets growing up. My grandmother used to eat them and they made me sick to my stomach! Now I love them on salads, in juices…actually one of my favorite things to eat. Beets are great for digestion and cleansing the body. But don't overdo it on the beets and always mix them with other fruits and veggies as they are a very powerful detox.

12 oz. green tea
Half of a small beet
1 small orange
1 inch piece of ginger
4 oz. cranberry juice
1 teaspoon stevia
1 handful of ice

Variation:

12 oz. chamomile tea
Half of a small beet
1 red apple
1 teaspoon stevia
1 handful of ice

Process ingredients in blender. Strain pulp using nut milk bag or sieve. Serve.

.....

Because beets do cleanse the body, don't be surprised if you get a headache after consuming beet juice. This is called a Herxheimer Reaction. Increase your water to help flush the toxins. It is a powerful superfood!

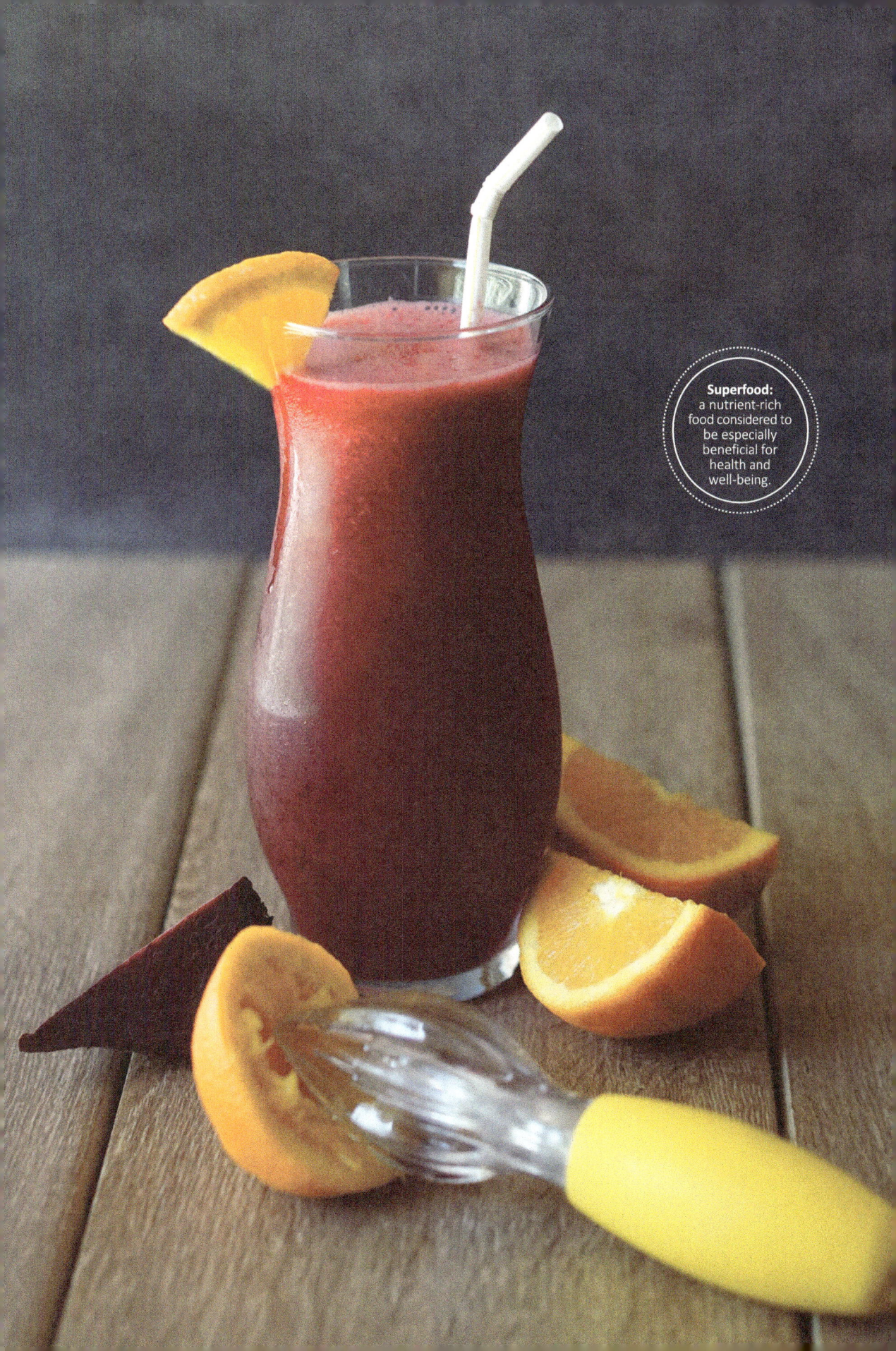

Superfood: a nutrient-rich food considered to be especially beneficial for health and well-being.

carrot juice

[Serves 1]

Many of us have heard about the benefits of carrots for eye health. But did you know that carrots are also known for helping to relieve congestion, fight inflammation, cleanse the kidneys? These spicy drinks will wake your body up and support your immune system.

12 oz. green tea
1 cup carrots
Dash of turmeric
1 small lemon
1/2 orange
1 inch piece of ginger
1 teaspoon stevia
1 handful of ice

Variation:

12 oz. chamomile tea
1 cup carrots
1 small lemon
1 red apple
1 inch piece of ginger
1 teaspoon stevia
1 handful of ice

Process ingredients in blender. Strain pulp using nut milk bag or sieve. Serve.

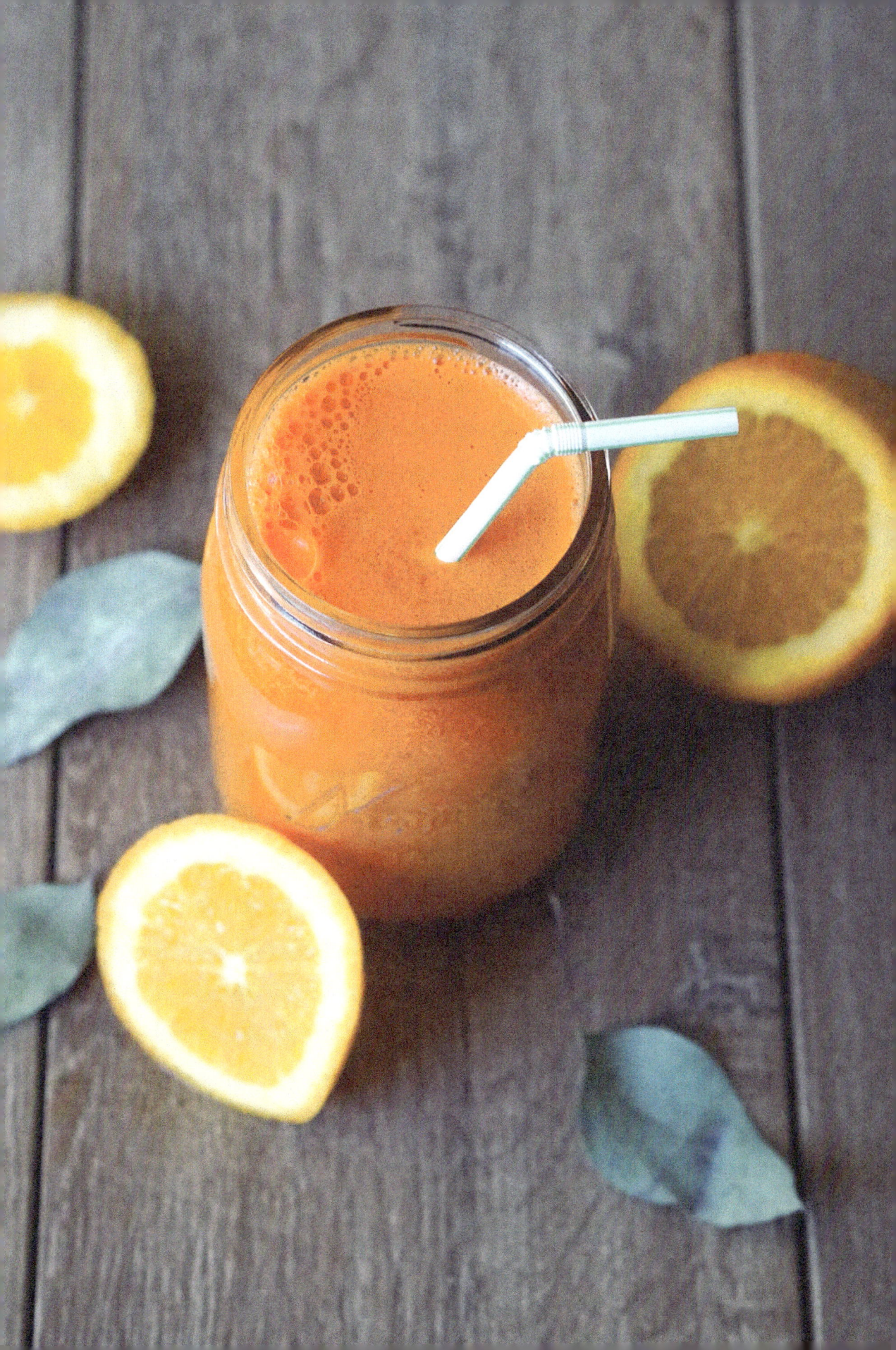

green drinks

[Serves 1]

Green drinks are packed with vitamins and nutrients that are good for you. However, if you are someone who suffers from oxalate kidney stones frequently or someone who is taking blood thinning medication, you will not want to consume too many green drinks, if at all. The oxalate in greens can cause kidney stones for some. And the high Vitamin K in greens can be problematic for individuals on blood thinners. Check with your doctor first, particularly if you are looking to do a juice cleanse.

Cucumber/Celery Juice:

12 oz. green tea
1/2 cucumber
2 celery stalks
1 small lemon
1 small green apple
1 teaspoon stevia
1 handful of ice

Collard Green Juice:

16 oz. green tea
2 collard green leaves
1/2 cucumber
1 small lemon
1 red apple
1 inch piece of ginger
1 teaspoon stevia
1 handful of ice

Spinach/Broccoli Juice:

16 oz. green tea
1/2 cup broccoli
Handful of spinach
1 cup kale
1 small green apple
1 teaspoon stevia
1 handful of ice

Process ingredients in blender. Strain pulp using nut milk bag or sieve. Serve.

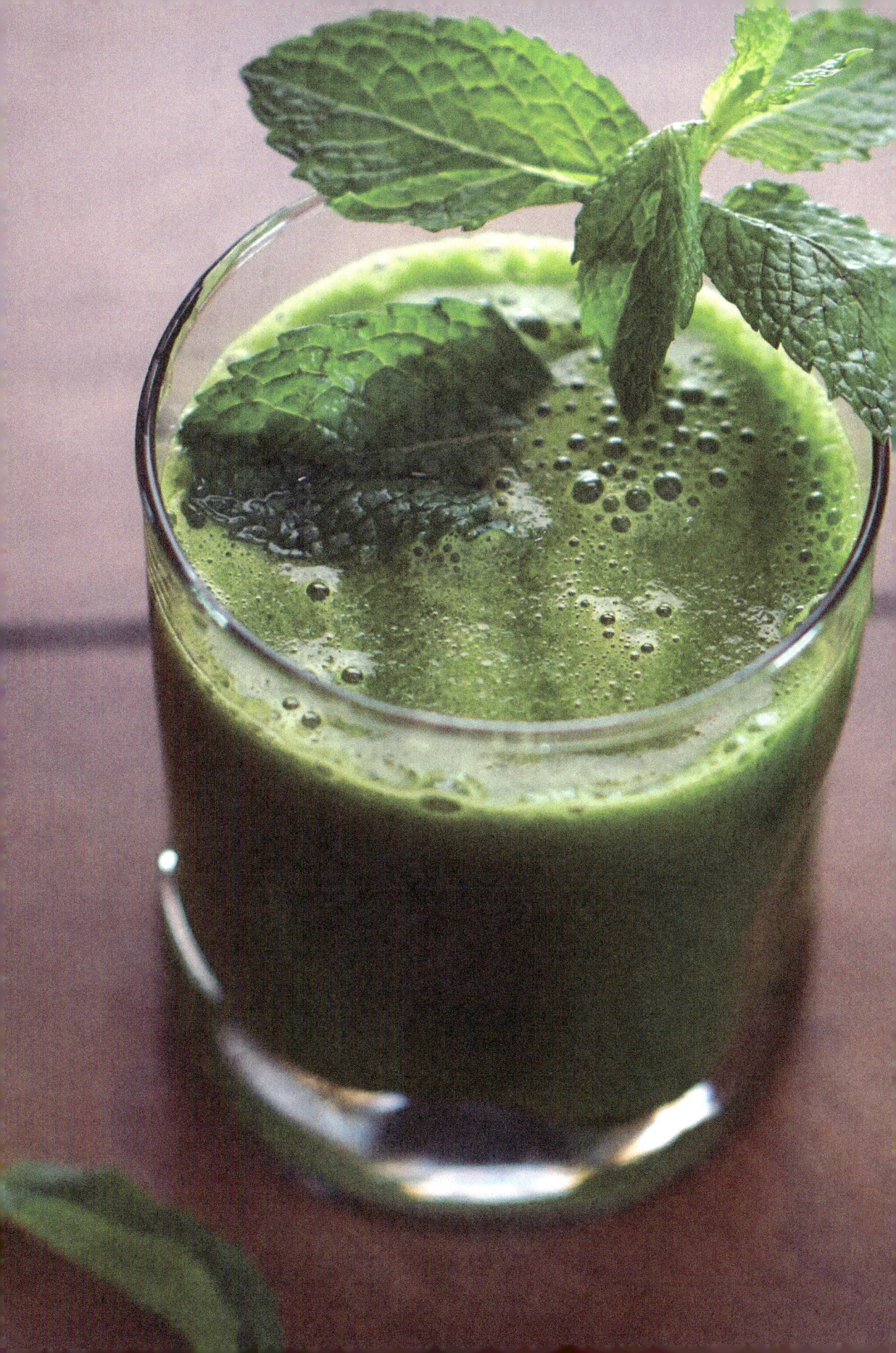

green drinks

[Serves 1]

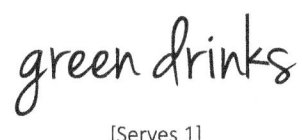

I love green drinks. I love the way they make my body feel and work optimally. And I actually love the taste! But the color and the vegetables make people cringe! Don't knock it til you try it! I use almost any green vegetable to juice with but my favorites are spinach, kale, collards, and celery.

Spinach/Kale/Parsley Juice:

16 oz. green tea
1 cup kale
Handful of parsley
Handful of spinach
1 green apple
1 kelp tablet
3-6 spirulina tablets
1 inch piece of ginger
1 teaspoon stevia
1 handful of ice

All Green Everything:

16 oz. green tea
1 small lime
1 green apple
Handful of spinach
2 celery stalks
1/2 cucumber
1 scoop green drink powder
1 teaspoon stevia
1 handful of ice

Process ingredients in blender. Strain pulp using nut milk bag or sieve. Serve.

.....
Boost your green drink by adding spirulina, kelp or green powder!

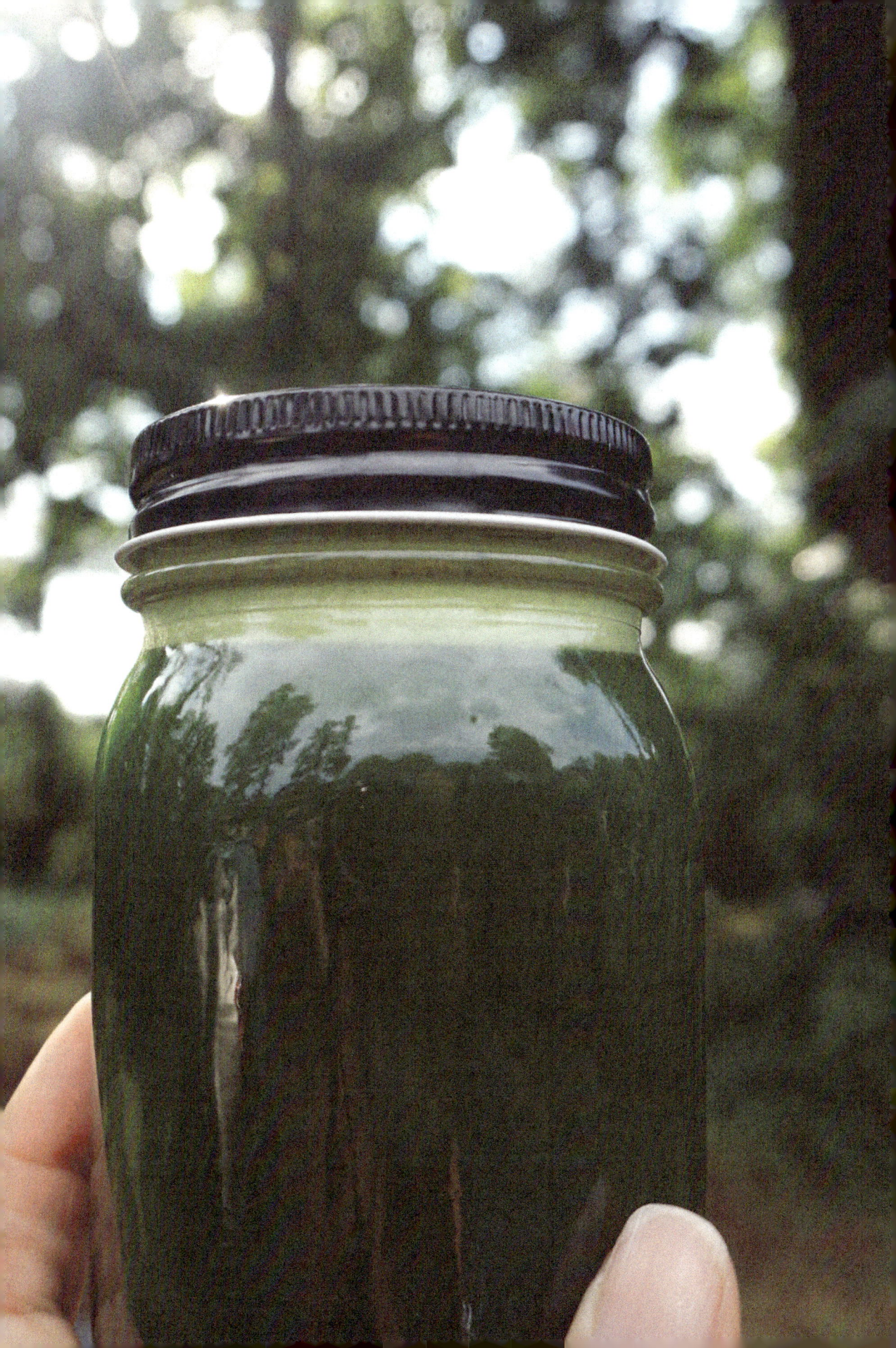

turmeric tea (hot)

[Serves 1]

This tea is a really warm and soothing drink. Good for aches and pains, digestion, inflammation and to promote relaxation.

1 ½ cup coconut milk
2-3 teaspoons of turmeric
Pinch of ground black pepper
1/2 teaspoon nutmeg
1 teaspoon cinnamon
1 teaspoon of powdered or fresh ginger
Stevia (or raw honey), to taste

Combine all ingredients, except the sweetener, in small saucepan. Bring to gentle boil without scalding the milk. Remove from heat and strain. Add stevia or raw honey and serve warm.

turmeric tea (cold)

[Serves 1]

This tea is a cool, refreshing tea that helps with inflammation as well as cools you off on a hot day.

16 oz. water
1-2 teaspoons fresh ginger
2 teaspoons turmeric
Dash of black pepper
One green tea bag, decaf
3 teaspoons stevia
1 organic lime

Bring water to a boil and add ginger, turmeric, a dash of black pepper, and a green tea bag. Turn off heat. Cover and steep for 5 minutes.

Discard green tea bag. Strain ingredients. Add stevia and stir until dissolved. Cool and add the juice of 1 organic lime. Add ice and serve cold.

.....
Turmeric stains everything it touches. So be careful to handle it with care. If you get a stain, a mixture of baking soda and lemon juice should get rid of it.

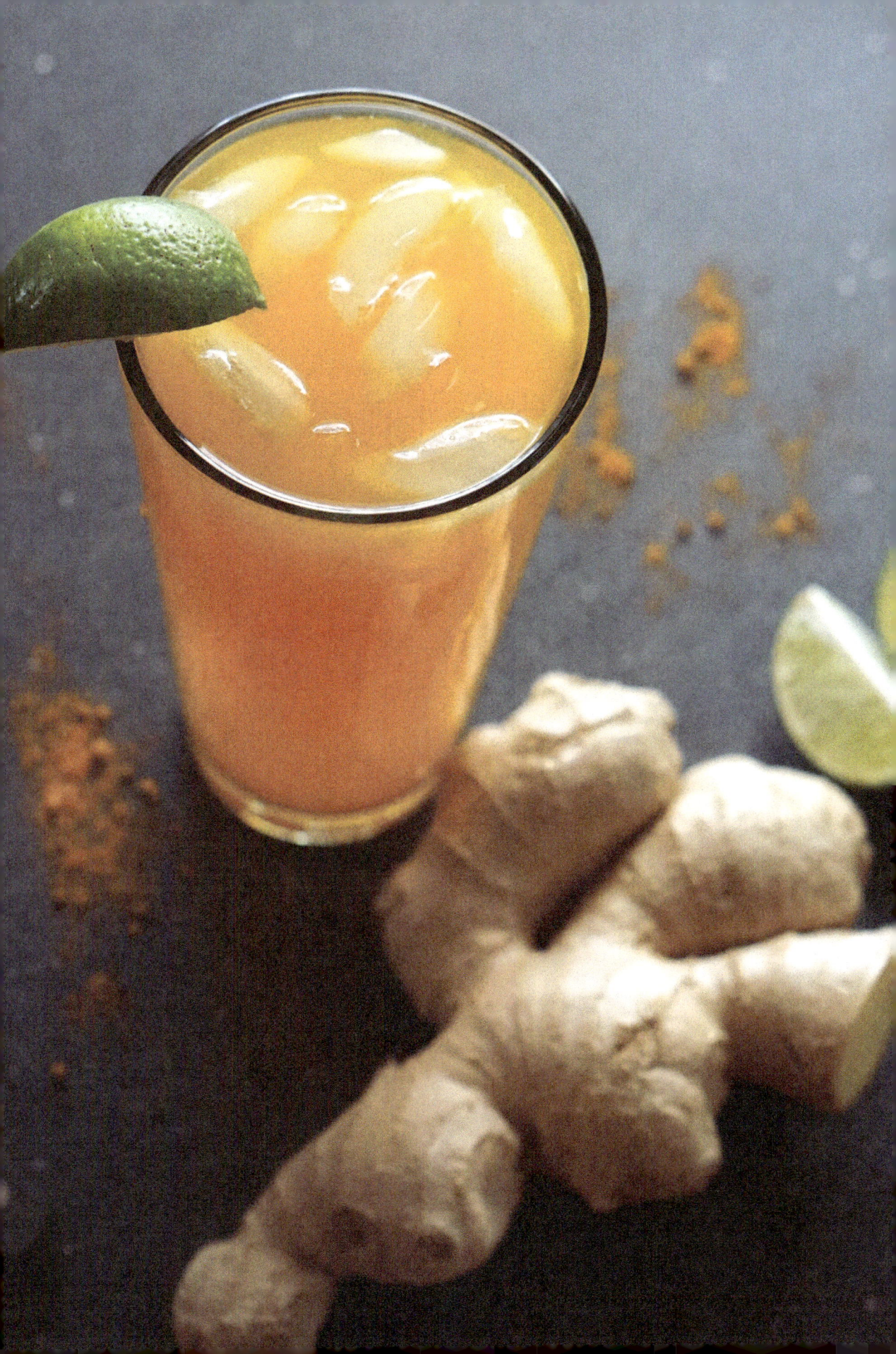

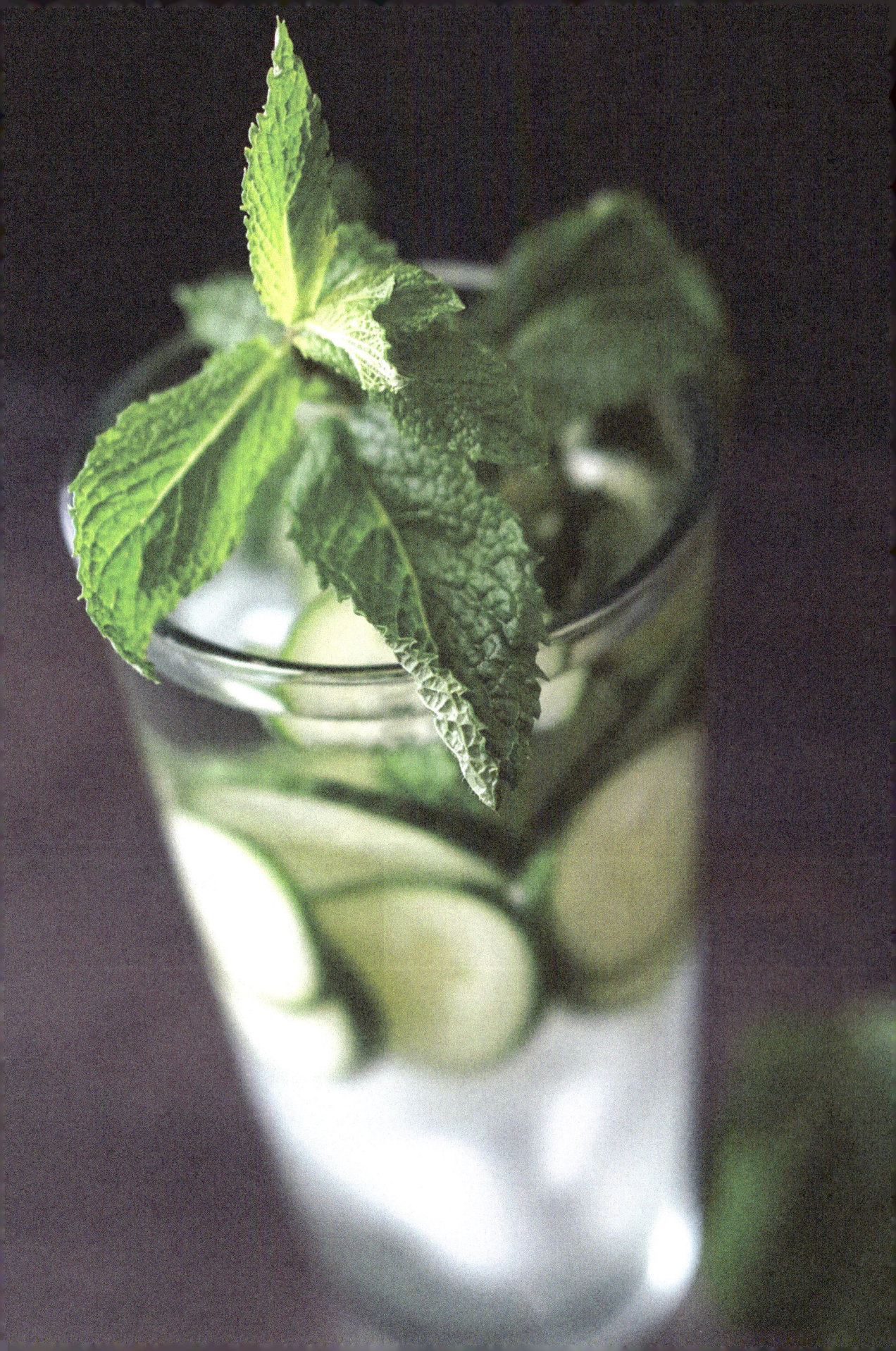

healthy mojito

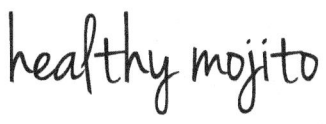

[Serves 1]

This cool, refreshing drink will quench your thirst and the infused water will also help detox your body.

12 oz. water (or green tea)
Juice of one small lime
1/4 cup cucumber slices
Handful of mint leaves

If using tea, brew tea and sweeten with stevia, if desired.

Pour liquid into glass and add fresh lime juice. Cut cucumber slices thinly and add, along with a handful of mint leaves.

Add ice. Serve.

.....
Invest in a fruit-infused water bottle so you can take your water on the go!

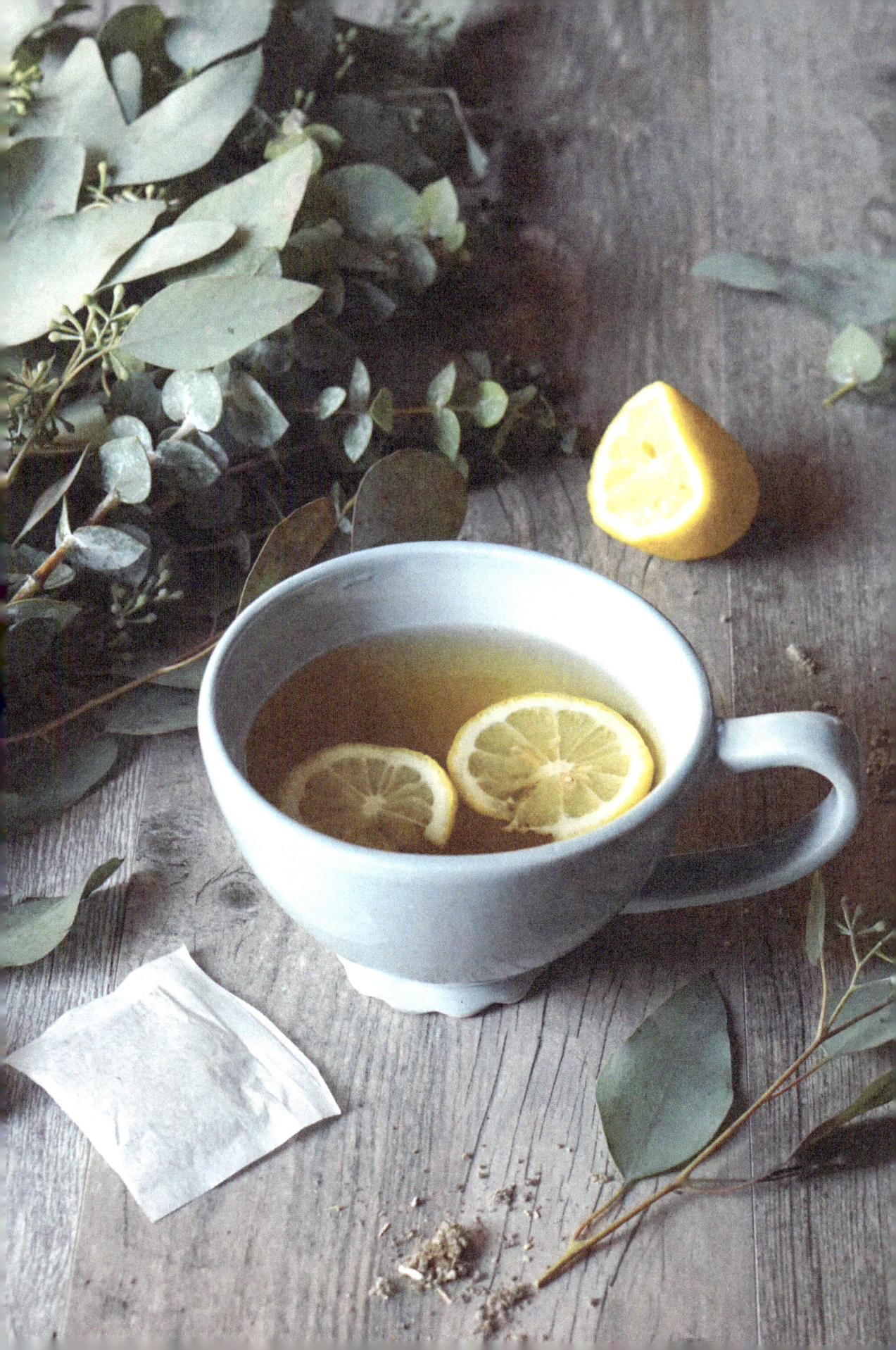

immune boosting drinks

[Serves 1]

Any time I feel a cold coming on, I go for one of these immune drinks. If I drink these 1-2 times a day, it will typically knock a cold out in an instant. Don't be afraid of the garlic. You might not be fun to be around for a few days but it does not taste bad at all...just adds a bit of kick to your drink. Garlic has anti-fungal, anti-bacterial and anti-microbial properties. It is a staple in my kitchen.

Hot Immune Tea:

1 garlic clove
1 ½ cups water
1 small lemon, cut into slices
2 inch piece of ginger
2 teaspoons organic apple cider vinegar
Raw honey, to taste

Crush garlic and let stand for 5-10 minutes. Boil water and add ingredients to the pot and steep for 10-15 minutes, with the exception of the honey. Remove from heat. Add honey to sweeten. Serve warm.

Morning Pick Me Up:

12 oz. green tea
1/2 pink grapefruit
1 small navel orange
1 inch piece of ginger
2 teaspoons stevia
1 handful of ice

Peel skin from citrus. Remove seeds from citrus fruits. Cut fruit into chunks. Process ingredients in blender. Strain drink using nut milk bag or sieve. Serve.

Cold Be Gone Juice:

12 oz. green tea
1/2 lemon, with rind (only if organic)
1/2 orange, with rind (only if organic)
1/2 pink grapefruit
2 inch piece of ginger
1-2 cloves raw garlic
2 teaspoons stevia
1 cup collard greens, kale or spinach
1 handful of ice

Remove the skin from the fruit and garlic. Cut fruit into chunks. Remove seeds from citrus. Cut greens and remove stems from the greens. Process ingredients in blender. Strain drink using nut milk bag or sieve. Serve.

.....

Be sure to smash the garlic before adding it and allow it to sit for 5-10 minutes so that the allicin is released, the compound that has the antibiotic properties to it.

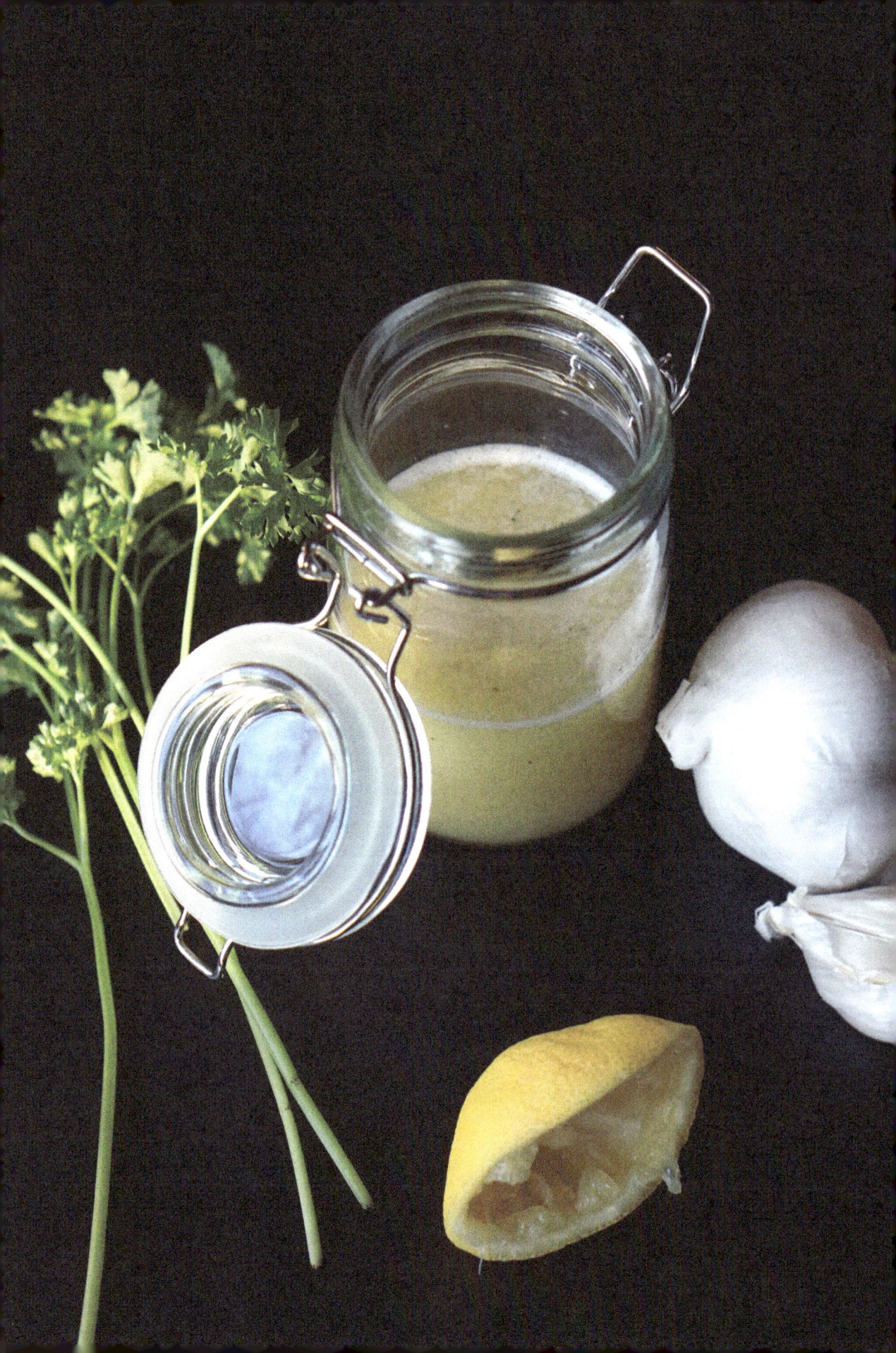

condiments

136 **Every Day Salad Dressing**
This is a quick and easy salad dressing that can be made in a blender or in a jar. Great on almost any salad.

137 **Poppy seed Dressing**
This poppy seed dressing is great on any fruit salad.

138 **Avocado Lime Dressing**
This is a creamy, tangy dressing that I love to pair with salads with strawberries or avocado. Also great as a topping for a burrito bowl!

140 **Mayonnaise**
No more hidden ingredients using store-bought mayo. Make your own at home in less than 15 minutes.

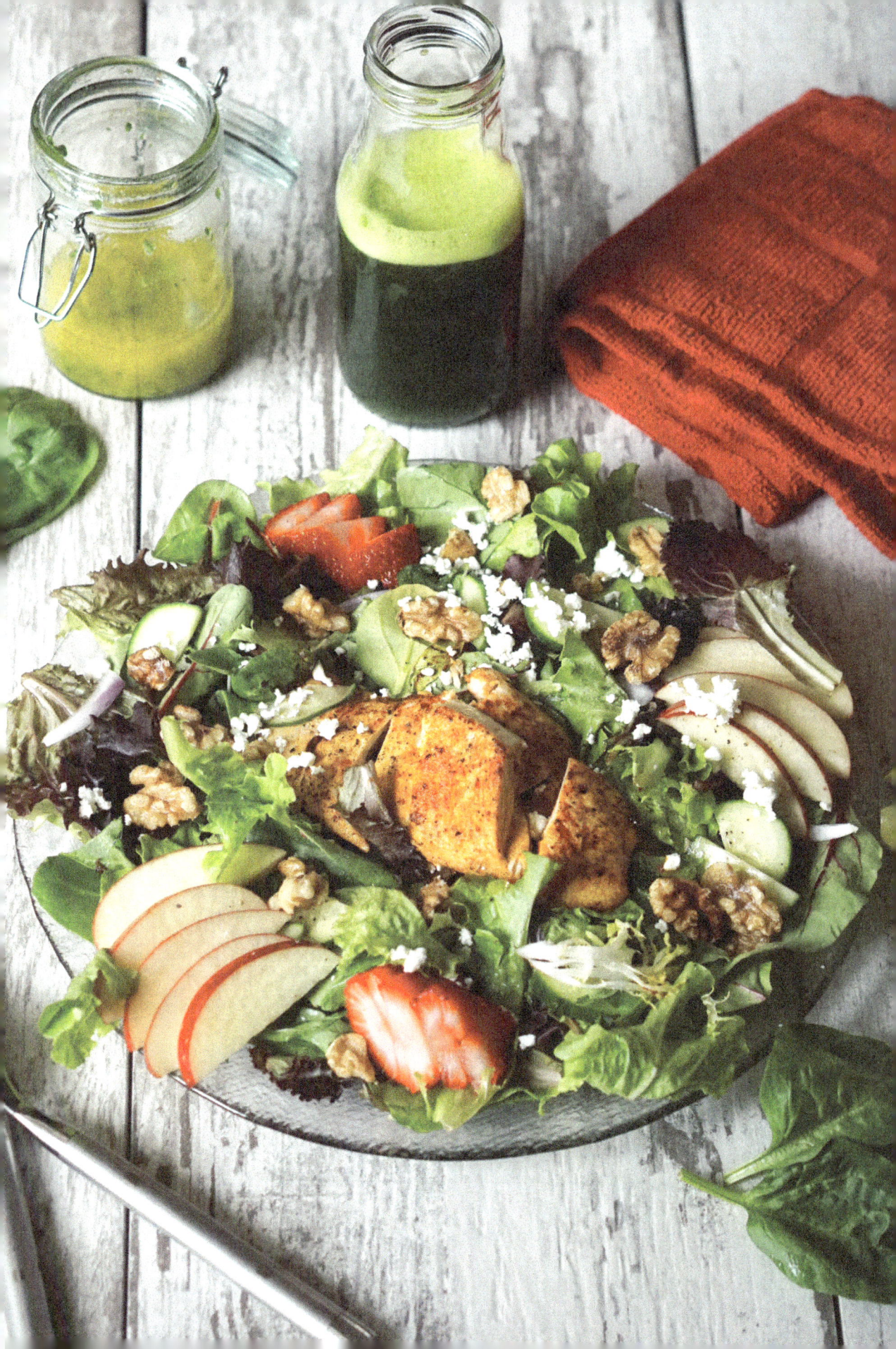

every day salad dressing

[Serves 4]

This dressing goes well on almost any salad and is easy to make. Can be made in a blender, with a mini food processor, in a bowl with a whisk or in a mason jar.

1/4 cup fresh lemon juice
1/2 cup extra-virgin olive oil
1 garlic clove
1 teaspoon stevia (or 2 teaspoons raw honey)
1 teaspoon fine sea salt
1/2 teaspoon freshly ground black pepper
1/4 teaspoon finely grated lemon zest, *optional*

Add all ingredients to a mason jar, blender or food processor. Process until smooth. Serve over salad.

poppy seed dressing

[Serves 2]

This is another favorite dressing that is simple to make and tastes good on almost any salad, particularly those with fresh fruits.

1/2 cup olive oil
3 tablespoons apple cider vinegar
1 teaspoon stevia (or 2 teaspoons raw honey)
1 tablespoon poppy seeds
1 teaspoon ground dry mustard
1/2 teaspoon ginger powder
1/2 teaspoon salt
1/4 teaspoon fresh ground black pepper

Add all ingredients to a mason jar, blender or food processor. Process until smooth. Serve over salad.

avocado lime salad dressing

[Serves 2]

This is a rich, creamy salad dressing that is delicious on salads, especially with shrimp, strawberries, avocado or salmon. This is also a great dressing on a DIY burrito bowl.

1/4 cup fresh lime juice
1/2 cup water
1 half of avocado, pitted and diced
2 tablespoons extra-virgin olive oil
1 teaspoon stevia (or 1 teaspoon raw honey)
1/2 teaspoon minced garlic
Pinch of sea salt
Pinch of ground black pepper

Add all ingredients to a food processor or blender. Process until smooth. Serve over salad.

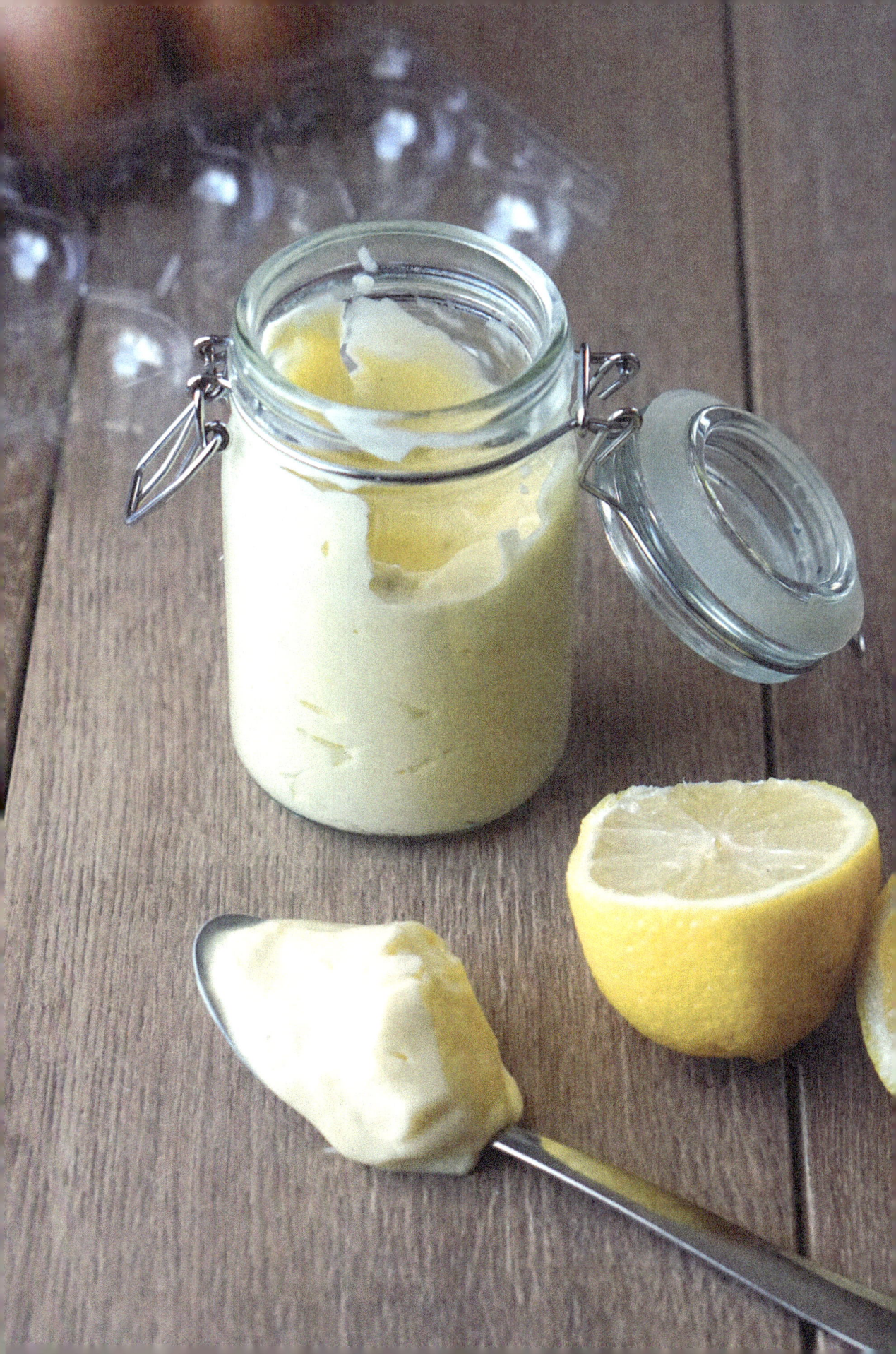

mayonnaise

[Serves 2-3]

I love tuna and chicken salad and while you can substitute coconut cream, along with apple cider vinegar, for a mayonnaise of sorts, I like having true mayonnaise on sandwiches and in chicken and tuna salads. Be careful not to add the oil too quickly or it will break and will not emulsify. Once you get the hang of it, you can do your own mayonnaise, baconnaise, or mayo with herbs.

1 Egg
1 Egg Yolk
2 teaspoons apple cider vinegar
1/2 teaspoon salt
2 teaspoons ground mustard
1/2 teaspoon stevia
1 cup avocado or grapeseed oil

Combine egg, egg yolk, salt, apple cider vinegar, ground mustard and stevia in a food processor. Start the food processor and add the oil very slowly, in the beginning.

Be careful not to incorporate too much oil initially or it will separate and you will have to start over. Continue to add oil in a slow stream until incorporated and the mayo is thickened.

Use within a week.

.....
Pasteurized eggs are safe to use in raw preparations - so be sure to use organic eggs to prevent risk of salmonella poisoning.

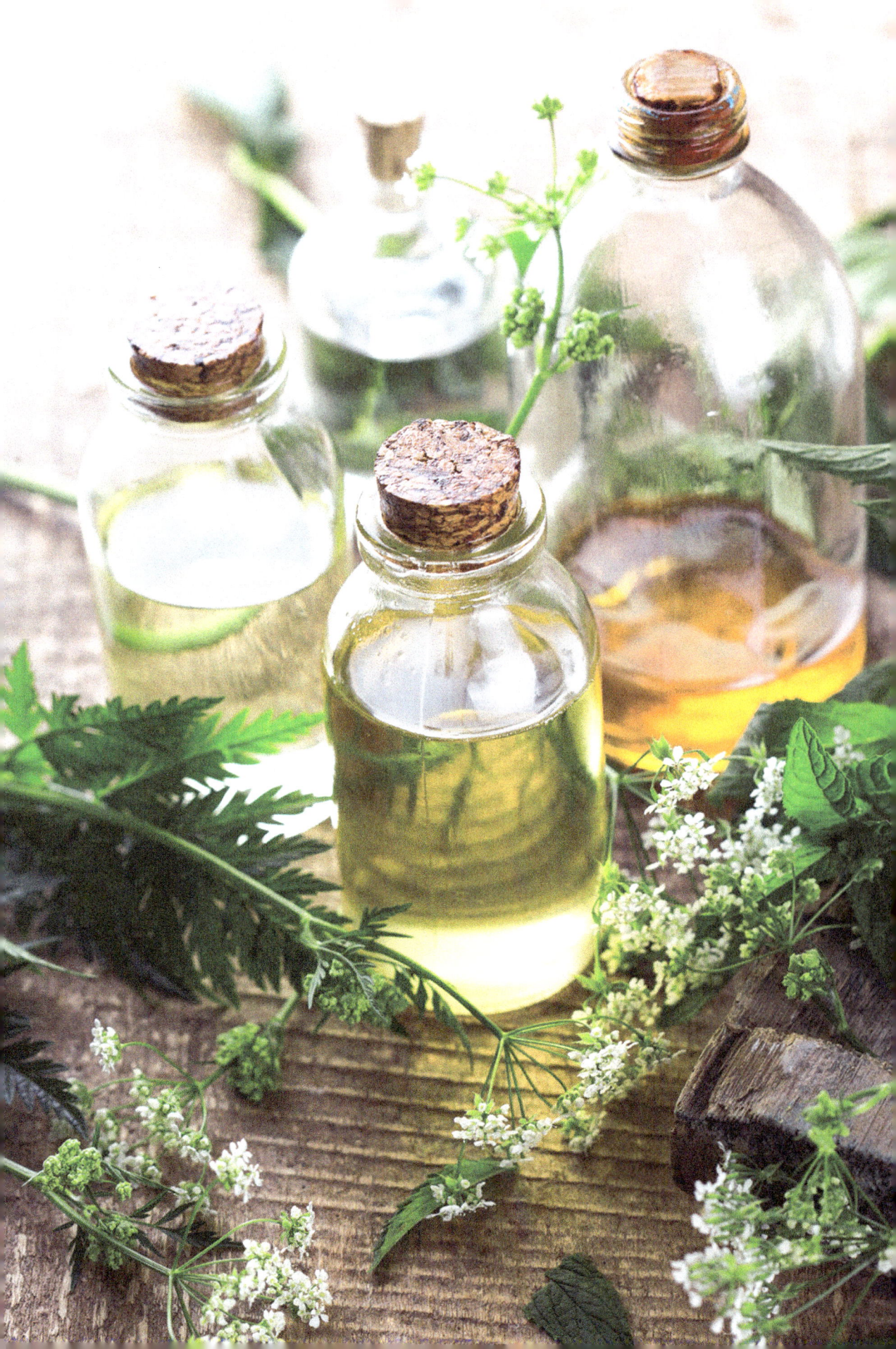

couple 'o extras

144 Detox Baths
When my body is toxic or when I am doing a cleanse, I add these detox baths to my regimen to sweat the toxins out more rapidly.

146 Dry Brushing
Enhance your detox baths, rid yourself of cellulite and get rid of toxins with dry brushing.

147 Oil Pulling
Try this ancient Ayurvedic remedy for detoxification and oral health. Improve your oral health with this simple, natural method.

148 Wet Socks Treatment
The Wet Socks method will help with sinus congestion and boosting the immune system. You can use the wet sock treatment to shorten the duration of a cold/flu virus, help with insomnia, and reduce fever.

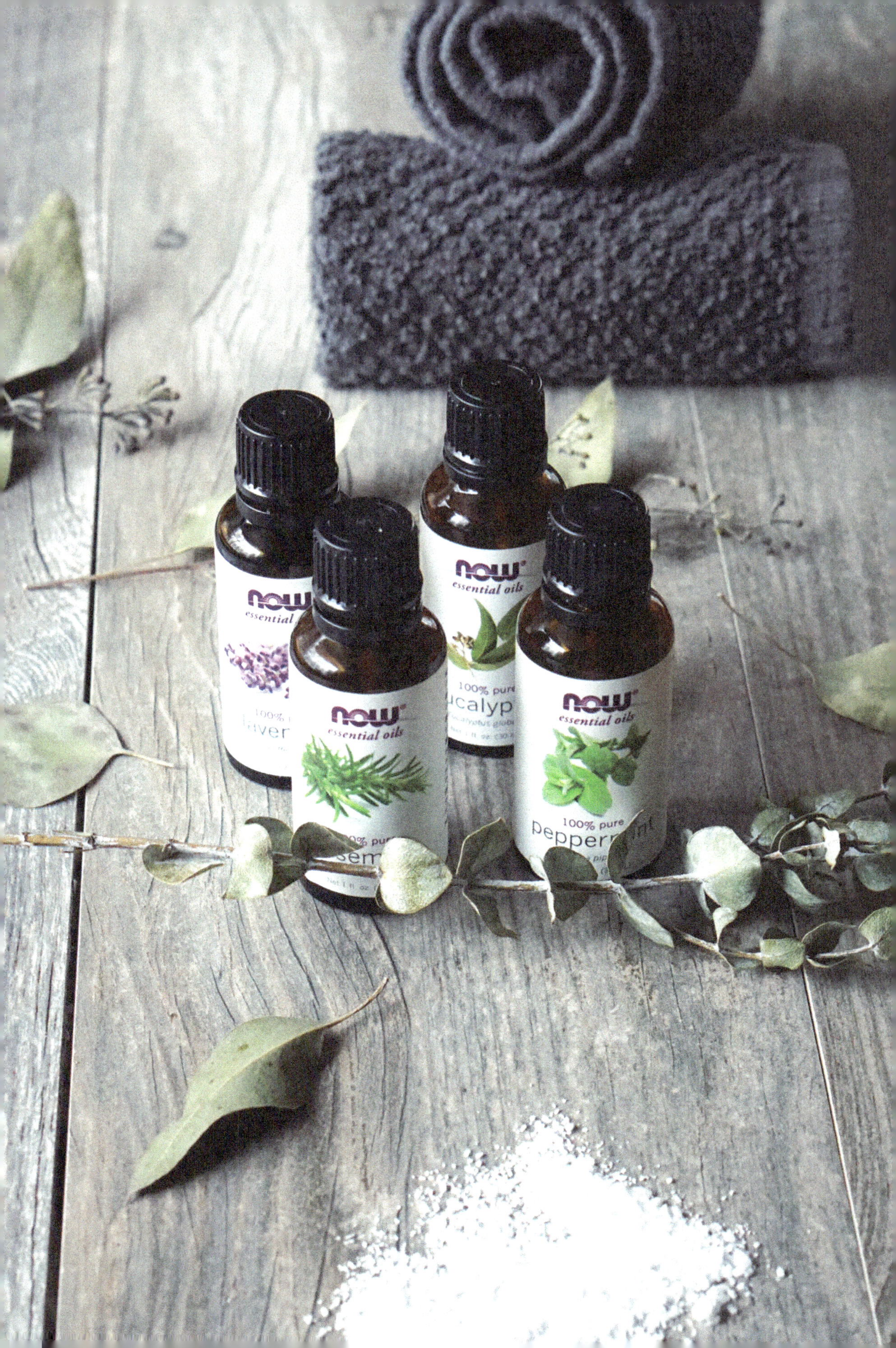
NOW
essential oils
100% pure
NOW
essential oils
NOW
essential oils
100% pure

detox baths

There are several different variations of detox baths but there are two that I use most often to sweat out toxins.

DETOX BATH #1
2 cups Epsom salt
10 drops essential oil

(Add Lavender and/or Peppermint for calming/relaxation; Eucalyptus and/or Rosemary for sinus/colds/flu/congestion, Tea tree for infection/rash/swollen joints)

DETOX BATH #2
2 cups Epsom salt
1 cup baking soda
2 ginger tea bags or
2 tablespoons ginger powder

Fill the tub with very warm water, as hot as you can stand it without scalding your skin. The purpose is to sweat out toxins!

Pour the ingredients into the tub and agitate the water to ensure they are dissolved.

Soak in the tub for 20 minutes.

Get out of the tub slowly. After sweating profusely and releasing toxins you may be dizzy.

Towel dry and rest.

TIPS:

1. You may sweat for a long time after you are out of the tub, which is normal, especially if you add ginger to the bath water. Therefore be sure to drink plenty of water before and after a detox bath to stay hydrated.
2. Do not eat a heavy meal after taking a detox bath.
3. You may feel fatigued after your bath. Therefore, I find that it is best to take a detox bath right before bed. It is a great way to relax before bedtime.
4. If you find that your heart rate begins to quicken while in the tub, slowly remove yourself from the tub or add some cold water to the bathtub.
5. *Optional:* Perform a dry skin brushing beforehand to remove additional toxins and then take your detox bath.

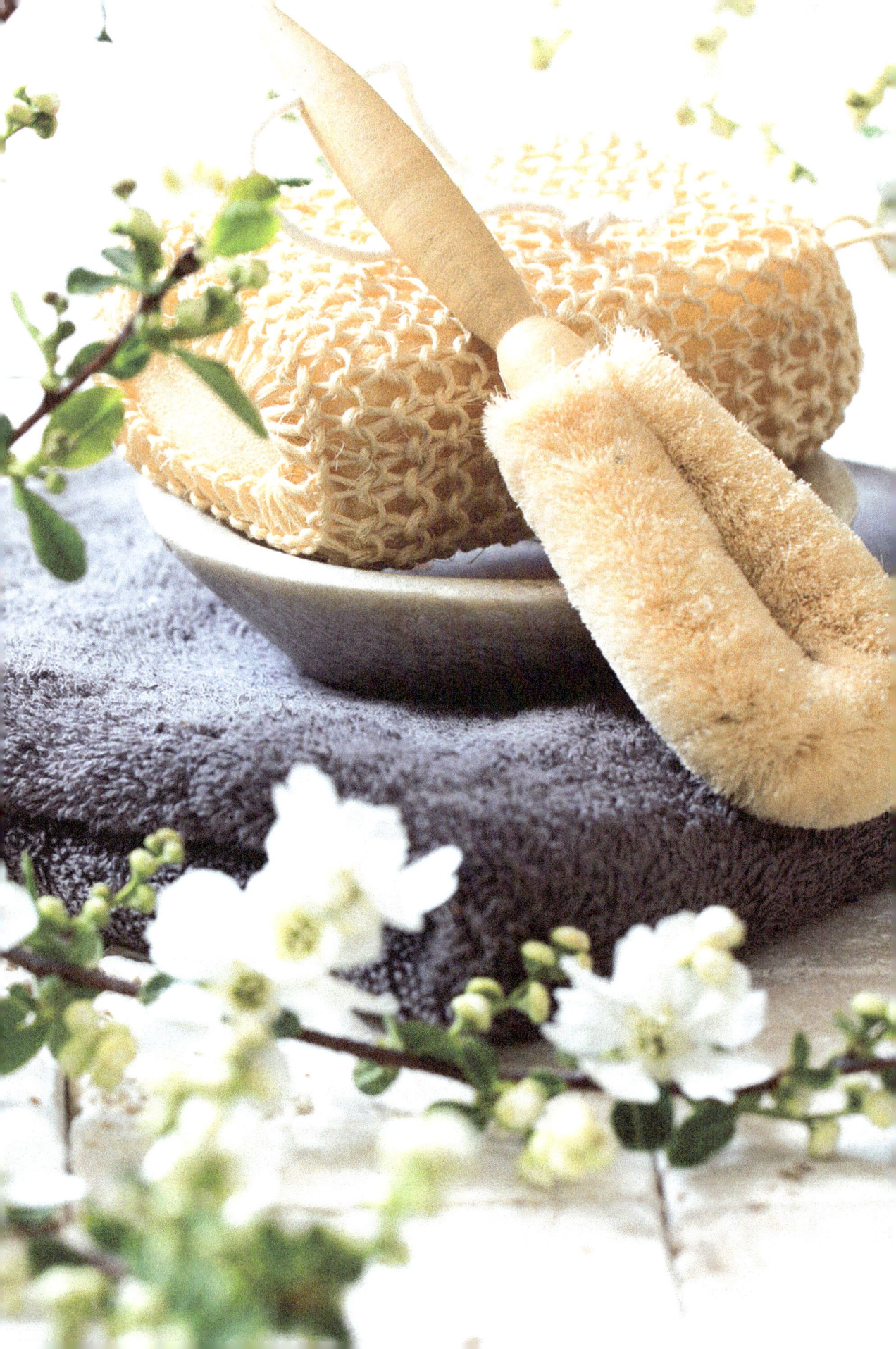

dry brushing

The skin is the largest detoxification organ in the body and serves as an elimination route for sweat and other toxins. Skin cells are constantly shedding and dry skin brushing helps facilitate the removal of toxins.

Dry Skin Brush

DIRECTIONS:
Always perform dry skin brushing before you shower so you can wash off impurities from the skin as a result of the brushing.

Start with a dry body and a clean, dry brush. Brush your entire body, from the soles of your feet upwards. Use long sweeping strokes in an upward direction to help drain the lymph back to your heart. Always brush towards the heart. When you get to the back, brush upwards on the back and down from the neck, again back to the heart.

Once you have brushed your entire body, take your shower as normal.

Be sure to hydrate the skin with lotion or coconut oil afterwards.

Benefits of dry skin brushing:

- Cleanses the lymphatic system
- Removes dead skin layers
- Strengthens the immune system
- Tightens the skin and removes cellulite
- Stimulates circulation
- Improves the function of the nervous system
- Improves digestion

Avoid sensitive areas and anywhere the skin is broken.

Use hydrotherapy to boost your lymph brushing experience. After you shower, turn on the water as hot as you can take it for several seconds, then as cold as you can handle it. Do this again for a few cycles to further invigorate the skin and stimulate circulation.

Clean your skin brush using soap and water once a week and allow to air dry before storing.

oil pulling

When most people hear about oil pulling they think it is insane...until they start going to the dentist and begin getting rave reviews about the vast improvement of their gums and teeth. Oil pulling is an ancient Ayurvedic remedy for detoxification and oral health. Science is now linking poor oral health to heart disease and systemic illnesses. So why not improve your oral health with this simple, natural method?

Organic Virgin Coconut Oil

DIRECTIONS:
In the morning, before brushing your teeth and on an empty stomach:

Take a teaspoon of coconut oil and swish in your mouth for 15-20 minutes (or as long as you can without swallowing the oil). Swishing will activate enzymes and the enzymes draw toxins from the blood. Do not swallow the oil, as it is now carrying the harmful bacteria from your mouth. Do not swish vigorously. Instead, slowly move the oil around your mouth so that your jaws do not tire quickly.

Once done, spit the oil in a grocery bag and dispose. Do not spit in the sink or toilet. One, it may eventually clog your pipes. Two, your mouth is full of bacteria so you don't want those toxins in your sink.

Rinse the oral cavity with warm water or warm salt water.

Brush teeth as normal.

Reported benefits of oil pulling:

- Whiter teeth
- Gingivitis and cavity prevention
- Strengthens the teeth and gums
- Clearer skin
- Less fatigue
- Decreased sinus issues

Note: Oil pulling is a detoxification method. As with any detox, as your body cleanses you may begin to experience a healing crisis or Herxheimer's reaction, such as headache pain, nausea, skin breakouts or acne...this is a sign that your body is cleansing. Those symptoms will not last very long so stick with it! If you get a headache, increase your water to help eliminate toxins faster.

wet socks treatment

My girlfriend went to see a naturopath who turned her on to this method to help with sinus congestion. I mentioned it to my naturopath and she advised me to use it as well to help boost my weakened immune system. You can use the wet sock treatment to shorten the duration of a cold/flu virus, help with insomnia, clear sinus congestion, boost the immune system and reduce fever.

1 pair of cotton socks
1 pair of wool socks
Tub of warm water
Ice Cold Water

DIRECTIONS:
Fill the bathtub with hot water (as warm as you can stand it without scalding yourself).

Drench the cotton socks in ice cold water (make sure they're saturated).

Soak your feet for 10 minutes in the warm water. *Note:* This method does not work if your feet are not warm. Once your feet are warmed up, pat them dry.

Wring the wet cotton socks to rid them of excess water. Cover your feet with the wet cotton socks. Immediately place the wool socks over the cotton socks and get under the covers and go to bed. TRY TO STAY UNDER THE COVERS.

When you wake the next morning, the cotton socks should be completely dry.

Repeat the wet sock treatment for three nights in a row for best results.

How it Works:

When your feet go from being hot to freezing cold, the body reacts to the cold socks by increasing blood circulation, which also stimulates the immune system. In doing so, it helps to decongest the upper body. It is also good for a very deep, calming sleep.

Do not use the wet socks if you have any open cuts on your feet, and be sure to check with your naturopath if you have any chronic conditions.

index

A

Almond 5, 7, 24, 28, 29, 34-35, 40-42, 44, 46, 49, 51, 56, 58, 67, 108, 112-113
    Almond Butter 5, 40, 44, 67
    Almond Milk 5, 24, 28, 34-35, 40-42, 44, 46, 112
    Almond Slivers 49, 51
Amino Acids 22, 24
Antibiotics 3-5
Apple 5, 22, 26, 35, 40, 42, 44, 48-49, 51, 53, 56, 61, 63, 71, 88, 92, 96, 102
    Apple Chips 102
    Gala Apple 26
    Golden Delicious Apple 40
    Rome Apple 26
Apple Cider Vinegar 5, 35, 53, 63, 71, 92
Applesauce, Chunky 96
Arrowroot Starch 5
Avocado 40, 42, 50, 59, 108, 138, 140
    Avocado Tart 1082

B

Baking Powder 28, 35, 115
Banana 46
Beans
    Garbanzo 99
Beets 58, 119
Berries, Mixed 110, 119
Beverages
    Beet Juice 119
    Carrot Juice 121
    Green Drinks 123, 125
    Healthy Mojito 130
    Immune Boosting Drinks 132
    Turmeric Tea 127
Black Bean 63, 74, 76
    Black Bean Burger 74
Blueberry 28
Bread
    Sweet Potato Bread 113
Breakfast 21
    Antioxidant Smoothie 41
    Apple Pie Smoothie 44
    Avocado Smoothie 42
    Blueberry Muffins 28
    Brown Rice Pancakes 34
    Fried Egg n' Hash 26
    Frittata 37
    Gluten-Free Pancakes 35
    Homemade Granola 29
    Kale Smoothie 40
    Parfait 32
    Quinoa Porridge 24
    Sweet Potato Smoothie 46
Broccoli 58, 67, 79, 123
Brown Rice 5, 34-35, 67, 74, 76, 81
    Brown Rice Pancakes 34
Brussels Sprouts 89
Buckwheat Flour 5
Burger 74
Burrito Bowl 76
Butter 5
    Butter Lettuce 73
    Butter Pecan 112
Buttermilk 5

C

Cake 115
    Lemon Pound Cake 115
Candida 4, 7, 11, 14
Canola Oil 71
Carrots 58, 67, 79, 81, 94, 121
    Rainbow Carrots 94
    Roasted Carrots 94
Cashew Butter 5
Celery 61, 63, 65, 71, 123, 125
Cellulite 146
Chamomile Tea 119, 121
Cheese 5, 7, 37, 49, 50
    Goat Cheese 5, 7, 37, 49, 50
Chicken 51, 67, 71, 73, 76, 79, 81, 83
    Chicken Apple Sausage 26, 61
    Chicken Breasts 20, 71, 76, 79
    Chicken Salad 71
    Chicken Stock 26, 59, 61, 63, 65, 78, 81, 92
    Roasted Chicken 51, 83
    Whole Chicken 83
Chips 102, 103
    Apple Chips 102
    Kale Chips 103
Chronic Fatigue 11
Chronic Lyme 16, 18
Cilantro 65, 76, 85, 97
Cinnamon 1, 20, 24, 34, 44, 46, 96, 102, 113, 127
Circulation 148
Clean 5, 7-10, 15, 18
    Clean Eating 5, 7, 8, 18, 20, 115
Cleanse 4-5, 58, 147
Clostridium Difficile (c. diff) 3
Coconut
    Coconut Aminos 5, 67, 73, 79
    Coconut Cream 5, 32, 65, 112
    Coconut Flakes 108
    Coconut Milk 5, 7, 42, 81, 108, 110, 112, 115, 127
    Coconut Oil 5, 28, 35, 91, 94, 108, 113, 115, 146, 147
Cold/Flu 123, 125, 132, 148
Compote 24
Condiments 133
    Avocado Lime Dressing 138
    Every Day Salad Dressing 136
    Mayonnaise 140
    Poppy seed Dressing 137
Congestion 148
Coriander 20
Corn 59, 76, 97
    Corn Syrup 7
    Roasted Corn 97
Cornmeal 78
Cornstarch 5
Cow's Milk 5
Cranberry Juice 41, 119
Cucumber 49, 51, 53, 59, 73, 85, 123, 125, 130
    English Cucumber 51, 59
Cumin 20, 26, 61, 63, 65, 74, 83, 94, 99
Curried Chicken 81
Curry
    Curry Powder 81

D

Dairy 3, 7, 18, 112
    Dairy Free 112

Desserts 105
    Avocado Tart 108
    Dairy-Free Ice cream 112
    Lemon Pound Cake 115
    Sorbet 110
    Sweet Potato Bread 113
Detox 4, 5, 9, 20, 58, 119, 123, 125, 130, 144, 146, 147
    Detox Baths 144
    Dry Brushing 146
    Oil Pulling 147
    Wet Socks Treatment 148
Dextrose 7
Digestion 4, 20, 40, 119, 146
Dill 53
Drinks 117
    All Green Everything 125
    Antioxidant Smoothie 41
    Apple Pie Smoothie 44
    Avocado Smoothie 42
    Beet Juice 119
    Carrot Juice 121
    Cold Be Gone 132
    Collard Green Juice 123
    Cucumber/Celery Juice 123
    Green Drinks 123, 125
    Hot Immune Tea 132
    Healthy Mojito 130
    Immune Boosting Drinks 132
    Morning Pick Me Up 132
    Kale Smoothie 40
    Spinach/Broccoli Juice 123
    Spinach/Kale/Parsley Juice 125
    Sweet Potato Smoothie 46
    Turmeric Tea (cold) 127
    Turmeric Tea (hot) 127
Dry Brushing 146

E
Egg
    Fried 26
    Fried Egg 'n Hash 26
    Yolk 34, 71, 140
Epsom Salt 144
Essential Oil 144
    Eucalyptus 144
    Lavender 144
    Peppermint 144
    Rosemary 144
    Tea Tree 144
Extracts 5, 115

F
Fajita 76
Flax Seed 24
Flour 5, 7, 28, 34, 35, 113, 115
    All Purpose (Gluten-free) Flour 35
    Almond 5, 113
    Baking 115
    Brown Rice 5, 34
    Buckwheat 5
    Coconut 113
    Sorghum 5
Frittata 37

G
Garbanzo 5, 63, 99
Garlic 26, 49, 56, 58, 59, 61, 65, 67, 69, 73, 78, 79, 81, 83, 89, 99, 123, 132, 138
Ghee 5
Ginger 67, 94, 119, 121, 123, 125, 127, 132, 144
    Ginger Powder 144
Gluten 7, 18
    Gluten-free 5, 28, 35
Goat Cheese 5, 7, 37, 49, 50, 51
Granola 29, 32
Grape Tomatoes 37, 53, 59
Grapefruit 58, 132
Grapeseed Oil 71, 140
Green Tea 119, 121, 123, 125, 127, 130, 132
Grits 5, 78
Guar Gum 112

H
Hash 26
Healthy Mojito 130
Hemp Milk 5
Herxheimer Reaction 5, 119
High Fructose Corn Syrup 7
Himalayan Pink Sea Salt 20
Homeopathic 15
Honey 5, 24, 29, 35, 42, 58, 127, 132, 136, 138
Hummus
    Red Pepper Hummus 99
Hydrotherapy 146

I
Ice Cream 110, 112
    Butter Pecan 112
    Vanilla 112
    Berry Sorbet 110
    Mango Sorbet 110
Immune System 3, 9 15, 18, 20, 121, 146, 147, 148
Inflammation 127
Insomnia 148

J
Jalapeno 63, 97
Juice 117
    All Green Everything 125
    Beet 119
    Carrot 121
    Collard Green 123
    Cranberry 41, 119
    Cucumber Celery 123
    Spinach Broccoli 123
    Spinach Kale Parsley 125

K
Kale 37, 69, 92, 103, 123, 125, 132
    Curly Kale 37, 61, 103
    Kale Chips 103
Kelp 39, 42, 125
Kidney 3, 5, 15, 20, 121, 123
Kosher Salt 20, 26, 53, 61, 71, 76, 78, 81, 83, 85, 89, 91, 92, 94, 103

L
Lemon 28, 115, 119, 121, 123, 132
    Lemon Juice 5, 56, 58, 71, 78, 89, 96, 99, 115, 127, 136
    Lemon Zest 28, 115
Lettuce 51, 73, 76
    Artisan Lettuce 51
    Butter Lettuce 73
    Lettuce Wrap 73
Lime 40, 42, 65, 76, 97, 108, 115, 125, 127, 130
    Lime Juice 59, 85, 110, 138
Liquid Stevia 29, 32, 56, 58, 67, 71, 110, 112
Liver 5, 15, 20, 58
Lyme Disease 3, 15, 16, 18, 20, 58
Lymphathic System 146

M
Mains (Lunch + Dinner) 47
    Avocado Soup 59
    Black Bean Burger 74
    Blackberry Apple Walnut Salad 51

Burrito Bowl 76
Chicken Salad 71
Cucumber Tomato Salad 53
Curried Chicken 81
Detox Salad 58
Kale and Lentil Soup 61
Kale Salad 49
Lettuce Wraps 73
Noodle Bowl 79
Pan Seared Salmon 85
Red Lentil Soup 65
Roasted Orange Chicken 83
Shaved Brussels Sprouts Salad 56
Shrimp n Grits 78
Stir Fry 67
Strawberry Avocado Salad 50
Turkey Chili 63
Zoodles 69
Mandolin 56, 102
Mango 85, 110
Margarine 5
Mayonnaise 71, 140
Mint 130
Molasses 7
Muffins 28
Mushrooms 37, 67, 78, 79, 92
Mustard Powder 56

N

Natural Remedies 144, 146, 147, 148
Naturopath 15
Naturopathic 15, 18, 147, 148
Navel Orange 132
Noodle Bowl 79
Noodles 69, 79
Nutmeg 24, 26, 44, 94, 96, 113, 127
Nutrition 15

O

Oatmeal 24, 44
Oats 29, 44
Oil Pulling 147
Oral Health 147
Orange Juice 46, 67, 83, 94, 113
Orange, Navel 132
Oregano 19-20, 74

P

Paprika 20, 61, 63, 71, 76, 81, 91, 92, 99
Parfait 32
Parsley 59, 61, 63, 81, 85, 97, 125
Peaches 56, 73
Peanut Butter 5
Pink Grapefruit 58, 132
Polenta 8, 78
Poppy seed 51, 71, 137
Porridge 24
Pound Cake 115
Protein 5, 9, 24, 40, 41, 42, 44, 65, 73, 79
    Pea Protein 5
    Whey Protein 5

Q

Quinoa 5, 24, 74

R

Raspberries 32
Raw Honey 5, 29, 42, 58, 127, 132, 138
Red Onion 37, 49-51, 53, 56, 58-59, 67, 71, 76, 78, 85, 97
Red Pepper 63, 65, 92, 97, 99
Rice 5, 7, 34, 67, 74, 76, 81
    Basmati Rice 76
    Brown Rice 5, 7, 34, 67, 74, 76, 81
    Brown Basmati Rice 76
    White Rice 5
Roasted Brussels Sprouts 89
Roasted Orange Chicken 83
Rolled Oats 44
Rosemary 20, 144

S

Sage 20
Salmon 85, 97, 138
Salsa 56, 76, 85
Saponin 24
Sausage 26, 61
Savory 26
Scallions 73-74, 76, 78-79
Seeds
    Pumpkin Seeds 29
    Sesame Seeds 29, 103
Shiitake Mushrooms 37, 67, 78, 92
Shrimp 67, 78-79, 138
    Shrimp and Grits 78
Sides n Such 87
    Apple Chips 102
    Applesauce 96
    Braised Spinach and Kale Medley 92
    Kale Chips 103
    Roasted Brussels Sprouts 89
    Roasted Carrots 94
    Roasted Corn Salad 97
    Roasted Red Pepper Hummus 99
    Sweet Potato Fries 91
Smoked Paprika 20, 63, 76, 81, 91
Smoothie
    Antioxidant 41
    Apple Pie 44
    Avocado 42
    Kale 40
    Sweet Potato 46
Snow Peas 67, 79
Sorbet 110
    Berry Sorbet 110
    Mango Sorbet 110
Sorghum Flour 5
Soy Sauce 5
Spices 20, 24, 74, 83
Spinach 42, 50, 92, 123, 125, 132
    Braised Spinach 92
Spirulina 125
Strawberries 32, 41, 50
Sucrose 7
Sugar 3-5, 7, 18, 29, 91
    Processed Sugar 5
Sunflower Oil 71
Superfood 49, 119-120
Sweet Potato 20, 26, 46, 61, 74, 91, 113
    Sweet Potato Fries 91
Symptoms 5, 8, 11, 15, 16, 18

T

Tahini 67, 99
Tapioca Starch 112
Tea
    Chamomile Tea 119, 121
    Cold Turmeric Tea 127
    Green Tea 119, 121, 123, 125, 127, 130, 132
    Hot Turmeric Tea 127
    Immune Tea 132
Thyme 20, 81, 83
Tomatoes 37, 53, 63, 69, 73, 76
Toxins 3-5, 9, 20, 119, 144-146, 147
Turkey 5, 63
Turkey Bacon 49, 56, 78, 89
Turkey, Ground 63, 73
Turmeric 20, 44, 46, 65, 121, 127

V
Vanilla Bean 112
Vanilla Protein Powder 40-42, 44

W
Walnuts 28, 50, 69, 71, 113
Wet Socks 148
Whey Protein 5
Whipped Cream 5, 32
White Sugar 7
Wrap 73

Z
Zucchini 69

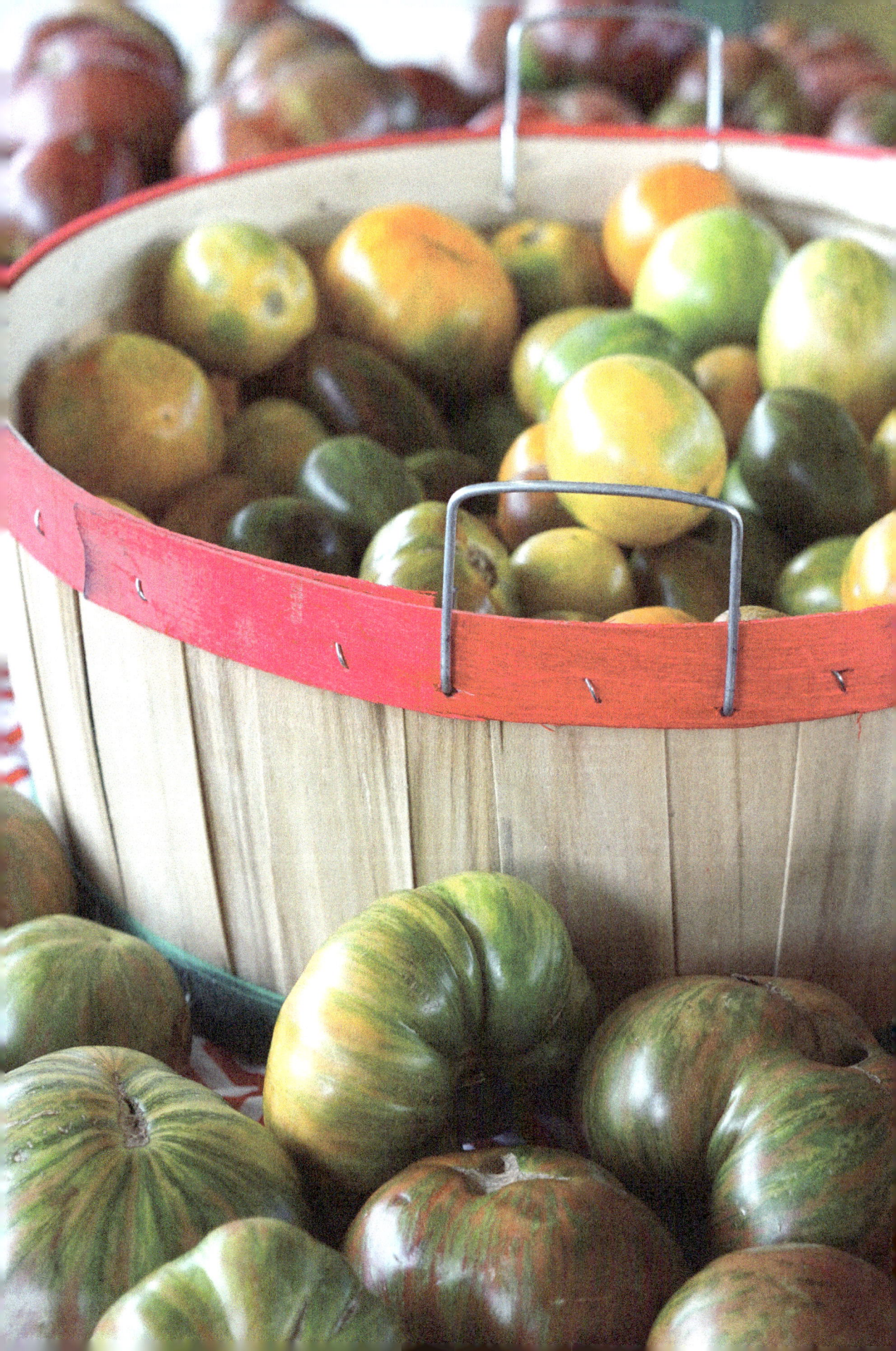

CPSIA information can be obtained
at www.ICGtesting.com
Printed in the USA
BVOW05*1813040517
483237BV00010B/33/P

9 780692 869642